AF711555

The Practical Assessment of Testamentary Capacity and Undue Influence in the Elderly

Eric G. Mart, PhD, ABPP (Forensic)
and
Adam D. Alban, PhD, JD

Professional Resource Press
Sarasota, Florida

Published by
Professional Resource Press
(An imprint of Professional Resource Exchange, Inc.)
Post Office Box 3197 • Sarasota, FL 34230-3197
Printed in the United States of America

Copyright © 2011 by Professional Resource Exchange, Inc.
All rights reserved

No part of this publication may be stored in a retrieval system, copied, scanned, reproduced, or transmitted by any means or in any form, except as permitted by provisions of the United States Copyright Act, without either prior written permission from the publisher or authorization (with payment of appropriate per-copy fees) from the Copyright Clearance Center, 222 Rosewood Drive, Danvers, MA 01923, (978) 750-8400, Fax: (978) 750-4470, E-mail: info@copyright.com, Website: www.copyright.com. Requests to the publisher must include precise written descriptions of (a) the material for which permission is sought, (b) the entity seeking permission, and (c) the intended use and circulation of the material if permission is granted. Requests to the publisher should be addressed to Permissions Department, Professional Resource Press, PO Box 3197, Sarasota, FL 34230-3197, Fax: (941) 343-9201, E-mail: permissions@prpress.com, Website: www.prpress.com.

This publication is sold with the understanding that the publisher is not engaged in rendering professional services. If legal, psychological, medical, accounting, or other expert advice or assistance is sought or required, the reader should seek the services of a competent professional.

The copy editor for this book was Patricia Rockwood and the managing editor was Laurie Girsch.

Library of Congress Cataloging-in-Publication Data

Mart, Eric.G
The practical assessment of testamentary capacity and undue influence in the elderly / Eric G. Mart and Adam D. Alban
P. cm.
Includes bibliographical references.
ISBN 978-1-56887-125-7
1. Forensic psychology. 2. Older people--Mental health. 3. Mental status examination. I. Alban, Adam D., date. II. Title.
RA1148.M293 2009
614'.15--dc22

2010019562

DEDICATION AND ACKNOWLEDGMENTS

This book is dedicated to the memory of
Maureen S. Mart
(10/18/1932 – 4/6/2009)

Dr. Alban would like to express his deepest gratitude to Tali, Alice, Scott, and Joshua for their unending support.

SERIES PREFACE

As a publisher of books, multimedia materials, and continuing education programs, the Professional Resource Press strives to provide clinical and forensic professionals with highly applied resources that can be used to enhance skills and expand practical knowledge.

All of the titles in the Practitioner's Resource Series are designed to provide important new information on topics of vital concern to psychologists, clinical social workers, counselors, psychiatrists, and other clinical and forensic professionals.

Although the focus and content of each title in this series will be quite different, there will be notable similarities:

1. Each title in the series will address a timely topic of critical importance.
2. The target audience for each title will be practicing professionals. Our authors were chosen for their ability to provide concrete "how-to-do-it" guidance to colleagues who are trying to increase their competence in dealing with complex problems.
3. The information provided in these titles will represent "state-of-the-art" information and techniques derived from both experience and empirical research. Each of these guidebooks will include references and resources for those who wish to pursue more advanced study of the discussed topics.
4. The authors will provide case studies, specific recommendations, and the types of "nitty-gritty" details that practitioners need before they can incorporate new concepts and procedures into their offices.

We feel that one of the unique assets of Professional Resource Press is that all of our editorial decisions are made by practitioners. The publisher, all editorial consultants, and all reviewers are practitioners and academic scientist-practitioners.

If there are other topics you would like to see addressed in this series, please let me know.

Lawrence G. Ritt, Publisher

ABSTRACT

This book is designed to provide mental health practitioners with a practical guide to assessing testamentary capacity and undue influence in the elderly. The first section provides an overview of the legal issues underlying such assessments as well as a guide to legal terms commonly associated with this area of probate law. The second section contains information on how to perform such assessments ethically and effectively. Specific information on the general methodology of such assessments, semi-structured interviewing, and appropriate psychological tests is also provided in this section. Case examples are offered to illustrate approaches to evaluations of testamentary capacity and undue influence. The CD-ROM included with this book contains a selection of instruments which may be employed by practitioners performing such assessments.

ABOUT THE AUTHORS

Eric G. Mart, PhD, ABPP (Forensic) received his doctorate in school psychology from Ferkauf Graduate School of Psychology in 1983. He then completed a postdoctoral retraining internship at the Pauline Warfield Lewis Center in Cincinnati, Ohio in 1986. Dr. Mart subsequently moved to New Hampshire to work for the Concord School District. He obtained his New Hampshire psychologist's license in 1987 and entered private practice the following year. Between that time and 2000 he obtained supervision in forensic psychology and became a board-certified forensic psychologist through the American Board of Forensic Psychology in 2002.

Dr. Mart's practice includes the treatment of children, adolescents, and adults; psychoeducational assessment, school consultation, and forensic psychology. His areas of forensic practice include the assessment of civil and criminal competencies, personal injury, child custody, and parenting assessments. He is best known for his work in the area of Factitious Disorder by Proxy (Munchausen's Syndrome by Proxy) and is the author of *Munchausen's Syndrome by Proxy Reconsidered.* He is also the author of *Issue Focused Forensic Child Custody Assessment* and *Getting Started in Forensic Psychology Practice*. In addition, he has written numerous articles for peer-reviewed journals and legal publications. Dr. Mart is past president of the New Hampshire Psychological Association. Many of his publications can be accessed at his website: www.psychology-law.com

Adam D. Alban, PhD, JD, is a clinical psychologist and attorney at law. He earned his MA and PhD from Michigan State University and interned at Western State Hospital in Tacoma, Washington. Dr.

Alban also has a law degree from American University's Washington College of Law. He is admitted to practice law in California. Prior to moving to California, Dr. Alban practiced in Washington, DC. While there he worked with adolescents, children, and their families throughout the District of Columbia on an individual basis, while also serving as a behavioral modification consultant to several schools. In addition, Dr. Alban functioned as a law clerk in the District of Columbia Department of Mental Health's General Counsel's office, where he worked at the nexus of law and mental health practice crafting policy, drafting regulatory changes, authoring legislation, and advising practitioners.

Dr. Alban currently resides in San Francisco, where he has a clinical/forensic practice. His forensic practice focuses on advising professionals who have fiduciary responsibilities on how to best serve clientele with diminishing cognitive abilities.

Dr. Alban also has a law practice that focuses on helping his clientele solve psychologically related legal problems. The majority of his clients are healthcare practitioners who have the need for legal services and advice incidental to their professional responsibilities. A frequent contributor to professional newsletters and other publications designed to serve the practitioner community, he maintains a database of these and other articles at his website, www.ClinicalLawyer.com, an online resource for clinicians. Dr. Alban can be reached via e-mail: alban@clinicallawyer.com

TABLE OF CONTENTS

The Practical Assessment of Testamentary Capacity and Undue Influence in the Elderly

INTRODUCTION

Testamentary capacity and undue influence are two areas in which forensic psychologists are likely to become increasingly involved in the coming years. This increase will almost certainly be driven by the aging of the "baby boomer" demographic, a group whose large numbers have had a major influence on the culture throughout their life span. In addition to the disproportionately large numbers of the boomer generation, this group is also relatively affluent and will have large amounts of money and property to distribute when they decease. This makes it likely that the number of legal challenges to their wills by those who are dissatisfied with the distribution of these assets will increase in proportion to the large numbers of elderly boomers who pass away.

Wills are contested for a variety of reasons. A common reason for such challenges is that the individuals bringing the challenge believe that they have been cheated out of their rightful inheritance through the underhanded maneuvers of the will's beneficiary. On the other hand, a concerned family member or friend may believe that the execution of the will is not an accurate representation of the testator's wishes, either due to lack of testamentary capacity or to undue influence. The combination of grief at the loss of a loved one, complicated family dynamics, and greed is a potent mix that can and does express itself through the litigation of the will in probate court.

The purpose of this book is to provide a concise guide to forensic practitioners wishing to provide psychological assessments and expert testimony to the courts in cases in which testamentary capacity and undue influence in wills, trusts, and similar legal documents are issues.

The first section, mainly written by Dr. Alban, will provide an overview of the legal context of these cases. Although this section is designed to help practitioners understand the psycholegal "terrain" of this area of probate law, it must be remembered that forensic practitioners have an ethical obligation to understand the laws governing these cases in their own jurisdictions. The next section is a collaboration between Drs. Alban and Mart and is designed to provide a methodology for assessing these types of cases, along with suggestions for techniques and instruments that can be utilized. In this section we have attempted to outline the nuts and bolts of performing assessments of testamentary capacity and undue influence. Included on pages 43-65 are a number of case studies that Dr. Mart authored, hence the use of the first person in that section. He has included analyses and reports (hybridized and altered to protect confidentiality) designed to take the reader step by step through the process of assessing, analyzing, and writing up reports in these matters. The CD-Rom that accompanies this book contains the Semi-Structured Interview for the Assessment of Testamentary Capacity (SSIATC) – an interview/information-gathering tool which both authors have developed to assist in such assessments. Also included on the CD-ROM are more assessment tools that can be used to aid in the assessment of testamentary capacity.

A WORD OF CAUTION

The assessment of testamentary capacity and undue influence, especially when performed retrospectively, is a complex and technical task. As will be discussed later in this book, the Ethical Standards and Code of Conduct of the American Psychological Association (2002) places special limitations on what can, should, and should not be opined by psychologists who cannot personally evaluate the subject of his or her assessment. To paraphrase the Standards, there is an obligation to inform the court and others involved in the case of the limitations imposed by these circumstances, including the need to rely on second-hand data and the absence of contemporaneous observations, interviews, and testing of the subject of the evaluation. This is an affirmative obligation and should be clearly stated at the outset of both the expert report and testimony; the expert should not wait for these limitations to be exposed through deposition and cross examination. Further, the Standards make clear that if there is not sufficient data on which to base a conclusion with reasonable certainty, then the expert should refrain from expressing an opinion. This is particularly important in retrospective analyses of testamentary capacity and undue influence, since there are cases in which medical records, unbiased personal accounts, or other necessary data do not exist. The expert in these cases should err of the side of not offering an opinion in these situations and avoid even the appearance of engaging in unsupported speculation.

This book is intended as a starting place for psychologists and other mental health professionals wishing to do these types of assessments. It will be important to review the available literature on the assessment of capacities and retrospective mental states to acquire a deeper understanding of the issues involved in such cases. Although many of these are mentioned in the bibliography, some deserve particular attention (i.e., Drogin, 2010; Grisso, 2003; Melton et al., 2007; Simon & Shuman, 2002).

Finally, in keeping with the requirements for competence laid out in the American Psychological Association Ethical Standards (2002), it is strongly recommended that mental health professionals new to this area of forensic practice seek consultation from an experienced colleague on their first few cases. This adds an additional set of safeguards to assure that the final product is accurate, effective, and performed in a manner that comports with applicable ethical standards.

DEFINING TERMS AND THE ELEMENTS OF TESTAMENTARY CAPACITY

Will contests and related proceedings typically take place in probate court. In general, *probate law* is considered separate from civil or criminal law. Black's Law Dictionary (2001) defines the term *probate* as "the judicial procedure by which a testamentary document is established to be a valid will; the proving of a will to the satisfaction of the court. Unless set aside, the probate of a will is conclusive upon the parties to the proceedings (and upon others who had notice of them) on all questions of testamentary capacity, the absence of fraud or undue influence, and due execution of the will." This means that, for practical purposes, courts assume that testators are competent to execute wills and that wills are free from undue influence and fraud. Moving each will through probate does not require a showing of competence and an absence of fraud and undue influence. Any party that wishes to dispute these three issues must raise them with the court. These presumptions of (a) competence, (b) lack of fraud, and (c) undue influence have implications for how these matters are evaluated, as we shall see below. First, however, a discussion of legal basics is in order.

WHAT IS TESTAMENTARY CAPACITY?

It is important to define the terms *testamentary capacity* and *undue influence* and also make clear what they are not. *Testamentary capacity* is best conceptualized as a type of competence, such as competence to stand trial or waive assistance of counsel. Testamentary capacity is essentially the minimum cognitive/emotional threshold the law requires an individual to reach before the law will recognize that a will is valid. This is an important legal act. All jurisdictions recognize the right of individuals to dispose of their property as they see fit (*American Jurisprudence* § 47, 2004). The states make laws that regulate this right, but as a general rule the right to dispose of one's property in a will is one that is protected wherever possible (*Hatheway v. Smith*, 1907). Even when under guardianship, many adults retain the legal right to make a will because the test for guardianship is different from the test for testamentary capacity. However, the previous appointment of a guardian may be considered as evidence in determining whether or not a testator was competent at the time a will was executed (*In re Estate of Kesler*, 1985; *Clement v. Rainey*, 1932; *Pape v. Byrd*, 1991).

Among nonlawyers and nonforensic mental health practitioners, testamentary capacity is sometimes confused with insanity, which is a different term of art. A term of art is a specialized way of using a word, with its meaning specifically defined by law. The term insanity in the law often refers to criminal capacity, which in its most basic form is the ability to determine right from wrong (*Slaughter v. Heath*, 1907). Testamentary capacity has also been compared to contractual capacity, though the two should not be equated in all jurisdictions (*American Jurisprudence* § 67, 2004). Competency to contract requires a meeting of the minds and the accompanying cognitive faculties, whereas testamentary capacity implicates the testator's ability to understand the functions of a will (*Slaughter v. Heath*, 1907). It is possible for an individual to not be able to conduct his or her ordinary affairs of business, but still be competent to construct and execute a will (*Singelmann v. Singelmann*, 2001). In many jurisdictions, these two competencies are distinct (*American Jurisprudence* § 67, 2004).

It is also tempting to link testamentary incapacity to the concept of mental illness, but this is a misunderstanding of what is required to execute a will. Though the inability to understand or perceive the functions of a will may be due to a major mental illness, psychopathology or cognitive impairment does not necessarily lead to incompetency (*Madden v. Cornett*, 1942). In 1981 the court held that although the testator had expressive and receptive language impairment, as well as a failing memory, other evidence showed that she was attuned to her surroundings and competent. She was able to recall critical information and communicated with her family, albeit slowly. The court rejected the argument that a specific diagnosis, by itself, was sufficient to establish incapacity (*In re Estate of Congdon*, 1981).

Thus ends our abbreviated discussion of what testamentary capacity *is not*. Understanding the legal theory of testamentary capacity in terms of the negative is useful because it helps evaluators to avoid "red herrings" that, though useful and occasionally promoted by one of the various parties, are not necessarily dispositive of this form of capacity. With this in mind, we now turn to the core elements of testamentary capacity.

THE ELEMENTS OF TESTAMENTARY CAPACITY

The question of testamentary capacity usually arises in two different circumstances. In the first, an expert is asked, either by an attorney or a family member, to evaluate an individual who is in the process of constructing a will (Melton, Petrila, Poythress, & Slobogin, 2007). In the second, an expert is asked to evaluate the competency of an individual who has already executed a will; in these circumstances the testator is frequently dead and this requires a retrospective evaluation of competency (Melton et al., 2007). In both of these circumstances, testamentary capacity is usually challenged on the grounds that the testator was either incompetent to execute a valid will or that the will was the result of undue influence. However, under both of these types of challenges, the question facing the court is somewhat similar: Did the testator have the capacity to execute the will (Frolik, 1999)?

The elements of the capacity required to execute a will are often addressed by individual state statutes. However, the requirements of many states have elements in common. These requirements are usually that the testator (a) knows the nature of the act of making a will; (b) understands the nature and extent of his or her property; (c) knows the natural objects of his or her bounty; and (d) knows how the will disposes of his or her property (Frolik, 1999).

Common Element #1: Does the Testator Understand the Nature of the Act of Making a Will? The first requirement indicates that those who are making the will or directing the construction of the will know the nature of what they are doing. This does not mean the testators must have an in-depth or sophisticated understanding of wills. It merely means that they are required to have a rudimentary understanding of the act of making a will (Melton et al., 2007). Testators should understand that, upon their death, the will transfers assets to the chosen heirs. An evaluator should establish that there were no delusional systems at work that were directing the testator's activity. For example, a testator who is constructing a will at the direction of intrusive thoughts or messages encoded in radio signals may not be directing the construction of the will. Evaluators can address this question directly to live testators in a structured or unstructured interview by asking them to explain items in the will and the rationale behind these provisions (Melton et al., 2007).

Common Element #2: Does the Testator Have an Understanding of His or Her Property? The second requirement is that testators should have an understanding of the nature and extent of their property, or at least the ability to recall this information (Melton et al., 2007). This is important because, in addition to the chosen heirs, the property is the focus of the will. But this is more than a test of memory (*In re Sixkiller*, 1934). If testators do not understand the nature of what they are giving away, they cannot be said to be making a reasonable decision regarding its disposal. The specificity of understanding required varies according to jurisdiction, but many states require that testators have at least a basic understanding that they possess key assets. Examples of key assets are items such as primary real estate holdings or significant investments.

When assessing this element of capacity, it need not be shown that, at the time the will was executed, testators recalled everything in their estate. More important is that testators had the ability to recall significant elements of their estate (*Holmes v. Campbell College*, 1926). Note that this also does not necessarily mean that testators must *appreciate* the size and contents of their estate (*In re Estate of Bennett*, 1993). Many wealthy individuals have complicated estates that are difficult to understand. Similarly, many individuals fail to manage their assets wisely. Competency does not require financial acumen, nor does it require an accurate recall of all the elements of an estate. In conducting an evaluation, experts look for a much lower standard. Evaluators should establish that, at the time the will was signed, testators had the ability to remember and understand significant parts of their estate. This is a fairly low standard.

Common Element #3: Does the Testator Know the Natural Objects of His or Her Bounty? A third requirement is that testators understand the natural objects of their bounty. This requires that testators know who are their natural heirs and the nature of these relationships. In some respects, wills are an alteration of the law's default position: The assets of the deceased are divided among the natural heirs according to statutory formulae. A will allows individuals to distribute assets according to their own wishes and to "opt out" of the statutory scheme. Provided that individuals have testamentary capacity, they are free to disinherit their natural heirs or to choose an unequal distribution (*American Jurisprudence* § 60, 2004). It should be noted, however, that some jurisdictions do not require testators to know who their natural heirs are (Melton et al., 2007).

Zorn v. Zorn (1933) presents an interesting perspective on the issue of natural objects of the testator's bounty. In this case the testator excluded one of his sons from his will. There was a history of acrimonious family relationships, and the disinherited son claimed that this history prevented his father, the testator, from understanding the natural objects of his bounty. Part of the jury instructions at trial read as follows:

> The aversion, dislike, anger, ill will and hatred, if such existed in the mind of said [testator] against his said son, must, in order to defeat the will, have been such as to overcome and control the will and dethrone the judgment of said [testator] in matters concerning his said son and must have existed at the time of the execution of the paper writing offered in evidence as his will. (*Zorn v. Zorn*, 1933, p. 626)

At appeal, the original beneficiaries claimed that this jury instruction was improper and the appellate court agreed, holding that "in order for ill will, dislike, or hatred toward a natural object of the testator's bounty to void a will, it must amount to an insane delusion existing without any reason or cause, however inadequate or unjust" (*Zorn v. Zorn*, 1933, p. 628). Because the conflict between the testator and his son was real and based on actual conflict, it was not an insane delusion. (A determination that a provision in a will is a product of an insane delusion is particularly significant because in many states such a determination invalidates the *entire* will.)

This application of the natural objects of bounty, though unsuccessful in this particular case, is instructive for experts conducting an evaluation. It indicates that cognitive distortions can affect several of the different criteria needed to establish competency. It is important for evaluators to address each of the different competency criteria in the jurisdiction and the ways in which perceptual and/or cognitive disturbances influence each prong of the test for competency. The requirement that testators understand the natural objects of their bounty is a prong that is in use by most jurisdictions. Evaluators conducting a thorough assessment should discuss the effects that cognitive and perceptual distortions have on testators' consideration and perceptions of their family.

Common Element #4: Does the Testator Understand How the Will Disposes His or Her Property? The fourth requirement is that testators are able to conceptualize the distribution of their assets and that they are able to demonstrate this by evincing knowledge of the plan for disposing of their assets. This does not require the testator to have a detailed understanding of how the assets are to be distributed, nor does it interfere with the executor's function. However, a rudimentary understanding is important, because the manner in which assets are distributed is a significant part of a will. The will is considered to express the wishes of the testator, and if the testator does not know how those wishes are to be carried out, the will could be said to not represent its author. If the testator is alive, he or she should be asked about the likely consequences of the property distribution. Who is to receive the testator's property, and is there a realistic understanding of how this is to take place (Melton et al., 2007)?

IS "REASONABLENESS" AN ELEMENT OF CAPACITY?

As noted above, testators are legally entitled to distribute their property as they see fit (*American Jurisprudence* § 47, 2004). If the testator was competent at the time of the will's execution, and the will does not violate any statutes, courts usually uphold its dispositions (*American Jurisprudence* § 59, 2004). This right extends to even unjust decisions and those to which no rationale can be applied (*Winter v. American Parkinson's Disease Association*, 1995). However, this is somewhat complicated for those assessing testamentary capacity, because an unreasonable provision in a will can be an indication of incapacity. Some provisions, such as those that assign property to nonexistent entities, may be a clear indication of incapacity (Melton et al., 2007). A provision such as "I leave my home to space aliens because my television has commanded me to do so" is unreasonable (*American Jurisprudence* § 75, 2004). But what indicates that the testator who made this provision may have been incompetent to do so is that the provision, according to its text, was not directed by the testator.

The line between a provision in a will that is so unreasonable that it indicates incompetence and a provision that is unreasonable without indicting the testator's competence is sometimes blurred. Several jurisdictions have allowed testators to leave portions of their estate to their pets (De Gale, 2003). Testators' wishes can seem unreasonable to those who are familiar with the testator, evaluators, attorneys, and even judges. When individuals struggle to understand the motivations of the testator, or perceive that the rationale behind the provisions of a will is unreasonable, the result can be a will contest.

For evaluators, the assessment question is not one of *reasonableness.* Fortunately or not, reasonability is not an element in the criteria for testamentary capacity. Evaluators should not use their subjective evaluation of reasonableness as an element in a capacity assessment. However, that does not mean that evaluators should refrain from using their clinical judgment of what is reasonable to inform their perception of a testator.

Unexpected, strange, or unreasonable items in a will are the clues that can reveal mental state (Melton et al., 2007). Thus, although unreasonableness is often important as a cue that assessment is warranted, evaluators should take care not to base their assessment on any reasonableness standard, because it is not part of the legal test for testamentary capacity.

In *In re Estate of Raney* (1990), experts testified that the testator suffered from a delusion that his family was working against him and that this delusion led him to believe that his family did not deserve any of his property upon his death. Experts also testified that although the testator was indeed suffering from a delusion, it was not so severe that it caused him to lose touch with reality. There were, in fact, verifiable conflicts between the decedent and the rest of his family, but the testator's perceptions of these conflicts were distorted due to the presence of brain damage and years of substance abuse (*In re Estate of Raney*, 1990). Medical experts testified that although the patient had a delusion, the delusion was not unreasonable because it was based in reality. At trial, the will was upheld. An appellate court agreed and rejected the challenge to the will. The Court made a distinction between delusions that are based upon *mistakes* and those that have no basis in reality. By declaring that the testator's delusion reflected a mistake, as opposed to a departure from reality, the Court validated the testator's will:

> An insane delusion is not established when the court is able to understand how a person situated as the testator was might have believed all that the evidence shows that he did believe and still [was] in full possession of his senses. There is no such thing as a delusion founded on facts or on a process of reasoning from facts. A person may harbor insane delusions and yet have testamentary capacity. A hallucination which indicates an overwrought imagination but not an impairment of normal testamentary capacity does not invalidate a will. (*American Jurisprudence* § 87, 2004)

This case and others like it have implications for experts who are assessing testamentary capacity. Strong convictions, even unreasonably strong convictions that border on irrational delusions, do not by themselves render a testator incompetent (*In re Kleeb's Estate*, 1982). Eccentricity or even bizarre behavior also does not, by itself, render a testator incompetent; the evaluation of competency must address how and whether the delusion affected the testator's ability to meet the requirements of capacity (*Applehans v. Jurgenson*, 1929).

This line of reasoning extends to distortions of perception and cognition that are caused by the ingestion of drugs. Wills that are executed while the testator is under the influence of licit or illicit drugs may be challenged on the basis of incompetency. Like challenges alleging that the testator was delusional, the moving party must highlight the nexus of perceptual distortion and testamentary criteria. The effects of substances must be such that they inhibited the testator's ability to competently execute a will. Testamentary capacity is a fairly low standard. Individuals with a drug addiction, even when under the influence, are not necessarily incompetent (*Smith v. Vice*, 1984). The same is true for individuals experiencing the effects of prescription medications (*Smith v. Vice*, 1984). For many people experiencing the effects of drugs or prescription medications, extreme impairment is episodic in nature. If a will is executed outside one of these episodes and at a time when the testator was lucid, the testator can be considered competent (*American Jurisprudence* § 73, 2004).

UNDUE INFLUENCE

An additional area of will disputes in which mental health experts are often asked to consult is the area of *undue influence*. Undue influence is a broader concept than testamentary capacity and arises in a variety of psycholegal contexts in addition to wills, such as contracts and prenuptial agreements. Undue influence is the substitution of the wishes of one person for another. In the context of the writing or modification of a will, the testator may, in the abstract, have testamentary capacity, but the wishes of another person are in fact what are represented in the will. In a claim of undue influence, the moving party requests that a will be invalidated, not solely because of a lack of sound mind, but because the effects of another person or persons were so great as to usurp the testator's free will (*American Jurisprudence* § 374, 2004).

An important conceptual distinction between testamentary capacity and undue influence is that incapacity is not an integral element of undue influence (*American Jurisprudence* § 381, 2004). Discussions of undue influence *assume that the testator had the requisite capacity to execute a will* (*Hamilton v. Morgan*, 1927), and "there can be no undue influence on a person devoid of mental competency" (*In re Estate of Anderson*, 1976, p. 587).

Yet, although testamentary capacity and undue influence are separate legal concepts, they are often considered concurrently. The Supreme Court of Arkansas has said:

> The questions of testamentary capacity and undue influence are so interwoven in any case where these questions are raised that the court necessarily considers them together, for in one case where the mind of the testator is strong and alert, the facts constituting undue influence would be required to be felt stronger than in another case, where the mind of the testator was impaired either by some inherent defect or by the consequences of disease or advancing age. (*Pyle v. Sayers*, 2001, p. 778)

In cases where a testator's will is constructed by and/or benefits another person, the issue of undue influence is often raised (*Pyle v. Sayers*, 2001). Note that it is not improper for influence to be exercised over an individual who is constructing a will. However, influence becomes undue if coercion or fear causes the testator to execute a will in a way that "constrains or coerces a person into doing that which his best judgment tells him not to do and deprives him of his free agency and substitutes the will of another person for his own" (*Kendrick-Owens v. Clanton*, 1999, p. 238).

THE PRACTICALITIES OF CLAIMING AND ASSESSING UNDUE INFLUENCE

Like testamentary capacity, the lack of undue influence is a rebuttable presumption in most jurisdictions. States assume that testators possess the capacity to execute their wills unless a claim states otherwise. Similarly, most jurisdictions assume that the individual who constructed a will was not under the undue influence of another at the time of its execution (*American Jurisprudence* § 371, 2004).

When the question of undue influence is raised, it is not uncommon for experts to be asked to assess the impact of disease and advancing age, as well as the degree to which these factors contributed to the alleged vulnerability of the testator. Mental health experts are often asked to evaluate the mental state of the testator, because showing that the testator's cognitive mental abilities were compromised can make it easier to successfully claim undue influence (*In re Brzowsky's Estate*,

1954). "The amount of influence necessary to dominate a mind impaired by age or disease may be decidedly less than that required to control a strong mind" (*Cook v. Huff, 2001*, p. 85-86).

WHAT MAKES AN INDIVIDUAL SUSCEPTIBLE TO UNDUE INFLUENCE?

There is relatively little literature in the mental health field about what exactly constitutes *a strong mind.* This is in part because *strong mind* is a legal concept. In contrast to other legal concepts that utilize information about an individual's mental state, literature on undue influence has not yet generated a corresponding scientific body of work (Marson, Huthwaite, & Hebert, 2004). This may be the case because mental state is only indirectly at issue in cases of undue influence. In cases of undue influence that utilize a mental health expert, the evaluator's testimony is often used to establish that, by virtue of a compromised mental state, the testator was unusually susceptible to the influence of another. Note that mental state in these cases is a *contributory* factor. Compare this to cases involving capacity, where the *primary* question is whether an individual's mental state itself prevented him or her from making a legal decision.

The available case law seems to indicate that the question of whether an individual has a *strong mind* is akin to the question of whether an individual is afflicted with a cognitive impairment. However, it may be possible that, in addition to possible impairments, the question of *strong mind* is one of personality. Personality traits such as *suggestibility* or the relative combination of traits such as *high-warmth* and *low-dominance* may also play a role in assessing an individual's vulnerability to undue influence (Gudjonsson, 1987; Morey, 1991). It is not yet clear if case law will eventually include personality traits as an indication of susceptibility to influence or if this will effectively lower the bar for claims of undue influence. Experts should be aware that standards for assisting the court with these claims are not yet fixed and may be largely dependent on jurisdiction and the legal theory pursued by the hiring attorney.

UNDERSTANDING YOUR REFERRAL SOURCE, AND WHY "UNDUE INFLUENCE" SOMETIMES REALLY MEANS "TESTAMENTARY CAPACITY"

As an additional practical matter, clinicians should be aware that undue influence is more likely than testamentary capacity to be raised in a will contest. The reason for this is that, in many jurisdictions, the threshold and accompanying case law that outlines a *prima facie* case for undue influence is much lower than that of testamentary capacity. In other words, to bring a postmortem will contest case alleging testamentary incapacity, an attorney must leap a fairly high hurdle. The same is not necessarily true for cases alleging undue influence. In many jurisdictions attorneys find it easier to make the initial case for undue influence. Because of this, clinicians may find that referrals that initially present themselves as questions of undue influence are actually questions about testamentary capacity. As discussed above, these questions are not entirely distinct, so it makes sense that there is some overlap. However, clinicians should consider having a discussion with referring attorneys to determine if legal procedural matters are clouding the referral request and, if so, whether a conversation to clarify would be helpful.

Considering the above discussion, the following potential indicia of undue influence should be considered in these assessments:

1. The accused party played an active role in procuring the will.
2. The accused party was in a confidential or fiduciary relationship with the testator.
3. The accused party unduly profited from the provisions of the will.
4. The presence of unnatural provisions in the will.
5. Provisions inconsistent with prior or subsequent expressions of the testator's wishes.
6. A relationship between the testator and the beneficiary that created an opportunity to control the testamentary act.
7. A mental or physical condition of the testator that facilitates subversion of the testator's free will. (Spar & Garb, 1992, p. 170)

There are other issues that can invalidate a will, and it is important to distinguish them from undue influence. One of these is fraud. Perr (1981, p. 16) notes that fraud "involves trick, deception and artifice; the testator is deceived by false statements or forged documents. False representations must be intermingled with importunities and attempts to influence to establish a claim of fraud. Fraud may be shown by a single act, while undue influence usually embraces a course of conduct." In the same way, duress is a concept distinct from undue influence which can invalidate a will. Duress has been defined as threat of harm made to compel a person to do something against his or her will or judgment; a wrongful threat made by one person to compel a manifestation of seeming assent by another person to a transaction without real volition. Duress involves the use of threats, force or other coercive behavior. An example of duress would be the use of blackmail to effect changes in a will.

THE ASSESSMENT PROCESS

AN OVERVIEW

There are many models which have been developed for forensic assessments, but few have been as influential and useful as Grisso's five-step model for the assessment of competencies (Grisso, 2003). This model describes five components that should be considered by mental health professionals assessing a wide variety of capacities. The model has the advantages of being simple but comprehensive; in addition, it allows the fact finder in the case to follow the methods and rationale of the examiner.

The first step in this model is the *functional* component. In this step, the psychologist gathers data designed to help determine whether the subject has or had the abilities required to perform the tasks involved in a specific area of competence. For example, in a competency to stand trial assessment, the examiner would gather information which would assist the court in its determination as to whether the defendant understands the adjudication process and can assist his or her lawyer in putting forward a defense. In a child dependency case, the functional component would be focused on whether the parent has the ability to adequately parent a minor. It should be noted that in some types of cases, a finding of adequate functioning may be all that is needed and there may be no need to pursue the other four components.

The next step in the model would be undertaken if deficits are noted in the functional assessment. Grisso (2003) refers to this part of the model as the *causal* component. This part of the assessment is designed to offer an explanation for any functional deficits noted in the subject's functional performance. For example, if a criminal defendant did poorly on tests related to competence to stand trial, the examiner would gather data designed to determine the cause of these deficits. An IQ test might be given to determine if subnormal intellectual abilities make it difficult for the defendant to understand the adversarial nature of a criminal proceeding, and other tests would be given to explore whether neuropsychological problems or mental illness play a role in functional deficits. It would also be important to explore whether underperformance or frank malingering play a role in the functional picture. A hypothesis-testing approach would be utilized to help explain the observed deficits.

The next component in the five-step model is referred to as the *interactive* component. This aspect of Grisso's (2003) model attempts to take the interaction between the subject's strengths and limitations and the environment in which they will be utilized into account. A particular defendant may have sufficient ability to participate in a simple assault trial in a local district court if there are only a few witnesses and the charges are straightforward, but may be unable to follow the proceedings in a drug sales case with multiple defendants, conflicting testimony and complicated legal standards dealing with intent. The interactive component provides the court with information about the subject's abilities in the context in which he or she will be called upon to use them.

The fourth component is what Grisso (2003) refers to as the *judgmental* component. This part of the methodology deals with the examiner's opinion on the ultimate issue in the particular case. For example, is the defendant competent? Can the mother effectively parent her child? Does the subject need a guardian? This component is controversial, because some authorities believe that such opinions are legal rather than scientific and that giving such opinions intrudes on the province of the judge or jury. Other experts believe that the judge or jury can give the opinion the weight they deem appropriate and are entitled to know what the expert thinks. If such opinions are provided, they should be limited and the basis of the opinion should be made clear.

The final component of this model is the *dispositional* or *remedial* component. This part of the model is designed to provide information to the court regarding the likelihood of the subject's functional capacity being restored. To use the example of competence to stand trial, a defendant who has functional deficits in his or her grasp of the issues involved in standing trial as a result of acute psychosis may be restored to competency through the use of antipsychotic medication. On the other hand, if the underlying cause of the observed deficits in capacity is the result of mental retardation or brain damage, there is likely to be less chance of restoration.

As previously mentioned, this model is flexible and can be used across a wide range of forensic evaluations. The model is applicable to the assessment of testamentary capacity and undue influence and will be utilized in this discussion of the assessment of these issues.

Before doing so, however, a discussion of the dynamic nature of competency is warranted. Witnesses and family members often have dramatically differing accounts of a testator's abilities. Of course, there is an array of explanations for such varying accounts, but a common (partial) task for evaluators is to account for and explain variability of functioning.

THE IMPORTANCE OF CONSIDERING VARIABILITY AND POSSIBLE IMPROVEMENTS IN FUNCTIONING

Because cognitive status fluctuates, competency also fluctuates. Thus, testators who are not competent to comprehend information about their will at one point in time may be able to process and comprehend this information at another point in time. For many testators with questionable capacity, decision-making capacity is erratic. Testators with some forms of cognitive impairment can be more or less alert, depending on any number of different situational variables. For patients whose cognitive functioning is acutely sensitive to factors such as nutrition, fatigue, familiarity of environment, or medication, evaluators should consider recommending that attorneys schedule appointments to coincide with periods of peak cognitive functioning. In the real world this may be somewhat difficult, and it may be appropriate for attorneys to have several conversations with their clients.

In many cases it may be possible to improve a testator's capacity. Although we are not aware of published studies examining the specific problem of improving testamentary capacity, there is an abundance of data demonstrating the effect of both instruction and situational variables on other adjudicative competencies. In the context of the criminal courts, competency to stand trial is often improved via treatment and instruction. The finding that competency to stand trial can be improved is robust. The construct of capacity to consent to medical treatment also has a rather large body of literature establishing its sensitivity to situational factors and "improvability" (Grisso & Appelbaum, 1995; Melton et al., 2007; Wong et al., 2000).

These data on capacity restoration seem to suggest that two promising methods for improving testamentary capacity are via (a) instruction, and (b) by altering the methods by which information about the testamentary instrument (or trust) is described to the testator. For clients with marginal capacity to understand the means by which the instrument manages their property, the most effective method for improving their capacity and ensuring that their wishes are carried out may be to provide the critical information in a simpler or altered format.

By way of example, some clients may be capable of making decisions and understanding the basics of their will, but be unable to appreciate the "usual" conversation that attorneys have with their clients. Busy attorneys sometimes have little time to educate their clients, and the rush to attend to the various demands of legal practice means that lawyers sometimes cannot spend as much time with each client as they would otherwise prefer. This is a reality of legal practice. Unfortunately, this can also mean that clients who are cognitively compromised face a barrage of complicated but very important information. For these clients, their competence may depend on an attorney's ability to "package" the necessary information in a more accessible format.

Borrowing from the literature on capacity to consent to medical treatment, one method of "repackaging" information would involve an initial complete disclosure, followed by a separation of the information into separate elements for separate discussion. This method might be best described as "repetition and staged disclosure" (Melton et al.,2007; Wong et al., 2000).

For example, a discussion between an evaluator and client would first require the attorney to articulate the essentials of the will.

Following this, the attorney/evaluator would then ask the client to paraphrase what the attorney said, and by doing so could monitor the client's understanding and rationale. Next, the attorney/evaluator would provide an accounting of the testator's property, following which the testator would be asked to paraphrase the information provided. This would then be followed by a discussion of the natural objects of the testator's bounty, and finally a discussion of how the will disposes of the testator's property (each of these elements would be discussed with an accompanying "check" on the testator's comprehension/ appreciation). Such an approach can be an effective means for simplifying a decision-making task for cognitively impaired individuals (Melton et al., 2007; Wong et al., 2000).

This is just one method for improving a cognitively impaired testator's capacity. Other methods can involve manipulating the situational variables to maximize alertness, such as by scheduling appointments at a time when the testator is maximally alert; for instance, before taking medications that may cause drowsiness or confusion. The central point is that evaluators and attorneys have a number of tools available to maximize testator competence.

Considering this, readers may want to consider the following recommendations:

1. Retrospective evaluations should include a discussion about the variable nature of competency, as well as data that supports a finding of competency/incompetency in and around the time in question.
2. Evaluators conducting a prospective evaluation should include data describing and explaining a testator's variability in functioning. Such a discussion can provide much needed clarity to attorneys (and courts) who are frequently faced with discrepant accounts of a testator's capacity

THE ROLE OF THE EVALUATOR

The performance of psychological assessments of testamentary capacity and undue influence will be discussed in situations in which the testator is alive, and also when the testator is deceased. The main difference between assessments conducted in these two situations is that it is not possible to use contemporaneous interviews, observations or testing in the case of a deceased testator, and greater reliance must be placed on other sources of data.

It should be noted that the Ethical Standards and Code of Conduct of the American Psychological Association (APA; 2002) addresses the need to be cautious and conservative in performing assessments when the subject of the assessment cannot be interviewed. The section of Bases for Assessments of the Ethics Code (section 9.01) states, "Psychologists base the opinions contained in their recommendations, reports, and diagnostic or evaluative statements, including forensic testimony, on information and techniques sufficient to substantiate their findings" (APA, 2002, p. 13).

This would seem to preclude performing assessments in cases in which the subject cannot be interviewed. However, the Code (APA, 2002, p. 13) goes on:

> (b) Except as noted in 9.01c, psychologists provide opinions of the psychological characteristics of individuals only after they have conducted an examination of the individuals adequate to support their statements or conclusions. When, despite reasonable efforts, such an examination is not practical, psychologists document the efforts they made and the result of those efforts, clarify the probable impact of their limited information on the reliability and validity of their opinions, and appropriately limit the nature and extent of their conclusions or recommendations.
> (c) When psychologists conduct a record review or provide consultation or supervision and an individual examination is not warranted or necessary for the opinion, psychologists explain this and the sources of information on which they based their conclusions and recommendations.

On a practical level, this means that it is ethical to perform an assessment of a deceased testator if the evaluator believes that there is enough information available on which to base opinions about testamentary capacity and undue influence. The evaluator should make clear any limitations that the lack of a face-to-face interview places on his or her data or refrain from giving an opinion if sufficient data do not exist. It should be noted that bringing out these potential limitations is generally considered an affirmative responsibility; such limitations should be brought to the attention of the fact finder at the outset of report or testimony. Having potential limitations brought out in the expert's report and in direct testimony serves two important purposes:

It helps to assure that the report and testimony comport with the aforementioned ethical standards, and also assures that the expert does not appear to be trying to disguise the limitations of his data.

There are situations in which a will may be contested before testators have passed away. This may occur because testators somehow inform interested parties of their intention to make changes in a will or when the parties otherwise become aware of some contemplated modification. In such cases, the probate court may order an assessment by a forensic psychologist or psychiatrist to help determine the extent to which testators understand the previously mentioned criteria (knowing the purpose of a will, that they are making one, a general idea of their property, the natural objects of their bounty, and the ability to keep all of these factors in mind during the making or modification of the will) (Melton et al., 2007; Wong et al., 2000). In preparing for such an evaluation, clinicians should review records so that they can assess the accuracy of the testator's answers regarding the property and assets and the structure of the testator's family.

In these cases, it is important for evaluators to clarify their role in the proceedings. Although this is always true in forensic cases, it is particularly important in cases involving testamentary capacity and undue influence. For example, the testator may be under a guardianship or medical power of attorney and may not have standing to consent to an assessment. In other cases, the psychologist may be approached by a family member to do an assessment when that individual does not have standing to request the evaluation. In these cases, it is incumbent on the professional to clarify the roles of the parties and make sure that performing the assessment will not lead to problems with multiple roles and other ethical entanglements.

For most mental health professionals working in this area of practice, the preferred way to come into these types of cases is as the court's expert, particularly when testators no longer have standing to give consent. An exception to this can occur when testators who are their own guardian request an evaluation of capacity prior to making changes in estate planning in order to head off an anticipated challenge to the validity of a will or related document. Assessments can also be performed at the behest of family members, and this is permissible as long as they have the legal right to have the testator assessed, although in these cases it is important to explain to the parties retaining your services that the assessment will be impartial and that your conclusions may very well run contrary to their desires in the matter.

THE ASSESSMENT PROPER

With the preliminaries accomplished, the psychologist can begin the assessment proper. The assessment should be performed in a setting that provides privacy and comfort for the subject. In some cases, testators can come to the psychologist's office, but in other cases they must be seen at their personal residence or at a nursing home. If the assessment is done outside the office, the psychologist should make sure a room with a table on which to work is provided. The testing room should be reasonably free of excessive noise or other distractions. The evaluation should begin with introductions and an explanation of the purpose of the assessment. This should be done even if the testator is not his or her own guardian; in keeping with the APA Code (2002) and the Forensic Guidelines (American Psychology-Law Society [APLS], 2008), a reasonable attempt should be made to obtain informed consent to the extent possible. If the testator is not his or her own guardian, it is important to obtain informed consent from the guardian prior to the assessment taking place, or at the same time if the guardian is present.

The issue of the presence of third parties in the testing room is controversial in forensic psychology. Some psychologists believe that third parties should be excluded for a variety of reasons, including the fact that the tests that are administered were not developed with third parties present. Others believe that as long as the observers are not intrusive, their presence is not a problem. Although there are valid arguments to be made for both positions, there are certainly cases in which the subject's comfort and confidence are increased by having a trusted third party in the room during the assessment. These issues should be approached with measured professional judgment on a case-by-case basis, but the authors generally do not object to an observer as long as he or she sits behind the subject's field of vision and does not speak except as indicated by the evaluator.

It is useful to develop a written agreement that specifies what type of evaluation the mental health expert is going to perform and the purpose of the assessment. The limits of confidentiality and the price structure of the evaluation should also be laid out, as well as any material required in the jurisdiction in which the evaluation takes place. Some professionals bill by the hour on these types of assessments. Others prefer to price these assessments by the job after they determine how much time will be required for direct assessment, record review, collateral contacts, and travel. In the latter case, the professional can name a figure and use the language "not to exceed" the amount quoted. It is important to note that the retainer should be received before the evaluation is undertaken and should not be contingent, as this could potentially bias the evaluator and is contrary to the dictates of the Ethical Standards and Code of Conduct of the American Psychological Association (APA, 2002).

Another issue that can arise is whether to record the interview. Again, opinions vary on the appropriateness of video or audio recording. The authors have come to the conclusion that it is best to create a verbatim record of the assessment, as this makes it possible for the court to make an independent assessment of our procedures and the validity of our conclusions. Also, there is a good deal of research that makes clear how inaccurate clinicians' notes can be and how much data is missed or misattributed. Videotaping is preferred, but can be cumbersome and complicated in certain settings. At a minimum, it is recommended that the clinician invest in a digital tape recorder that allows uploading of files to a computer so that CDs or DVDs can be made.

Another possibility is to use a product called the *Pulse Smartpen* (http://www.livescribe.com). This is a combination pen and digital recorder. It is used with special microdot paper which can be printed by the user or purchased from the manufacturer. As the evaluator takes notes, the pen records the interview. Later, if the evaluator wishes to know exactly what was said when a note was made, he or she simply touches the pen to the appropriate line and the recording starts at the point the note was made. This method of preserving the interview may be useful in that it is less obtrusive than setting up a video camera or placing a digital recorder on the testing table.

Assessment of the functional component of testamentary capacity of a living testator should include both a formal mental status examination and a clinical interview. The mental status evaluation provides the clinician with basic information regarding the testator's cognitive and emotional functioning which can then be provided to the court. The clinical interview allows the clinician to ask direct questions about testators' knowledge of the purpose of a will, the extent of their assets, and their rationale for their decisions regarding their distribution. Because the legal bar for testamentary capacity has traditionally not been set high, it is not necessary that testators know their assets to the penny, and the clinician should not hesitate to prompt subjects about specific assets that they may have temporarily forgotten. However, having prompted the subject, clinicians should revisit the material later in the interview to discover whether the information has been retained by the subject. (See the Frontal Assessment Battery (FAB), the Hopemont Capacity Assessment Interview (HCAI), the Informant Questionnaire on Cognitive Decline in the Elderly (IQCODE), and the Montreal Cognitive Assessment (MoCA) on the CD-Rom.)

If no significant deficits are noted during the functional assessment, this is often as far as the clinician needs to proceed. As with other competencies, when the subject is found to be able to demonstrate the requisite capacities, the referral question has been answered and no further information is required. However, in some cases it may be helpful to perform some testing when it has been suggested that there are cognitive or emotional deficits present, simply to provide a more complete picture of the testator's mental condition.

In circumstances where the testator is deceased, the clinician should carefully review the medical records of the subject in order to obtain information about the subject's mental state at the time the will was executed or when changes were made. Nursing notes and medical reports may indicate that the subject's emotional and cognitive functioning was reasonably good, or it may be revealed that there were major problems in one or both of these areas, such that serious doubts are raised about the subject's ability to grasp the issues involved in making or changing a will. The records may show a series of mental status examination administrations or Clock Drawings (Shulman & Feinstein, 2003) which were indicative of serious deficits in orientation and memory, and nursing notes may indicate that the testator was seriously depressed or psychotic, unable to perform activities of daily living (ADLs), or otherwise grossly impaired in functioning (Shulman & Feinstein, 2003). It can be helpful to develop a timeline with issues related to mental state on one side and the changes made to the will on the other. This allows the court to have a better idea of the sequence of events related to the will. A sample timeline is shown in Figure 1 (p. 25). (Also see the Retrospective Form of the IQCODE on the CD-Rom.)

If deficits in the functional ability to make a will are detected, the evaluator would then move on to address the causal component as suggested in the five-step model (Grisso, 2003). In this phase, the

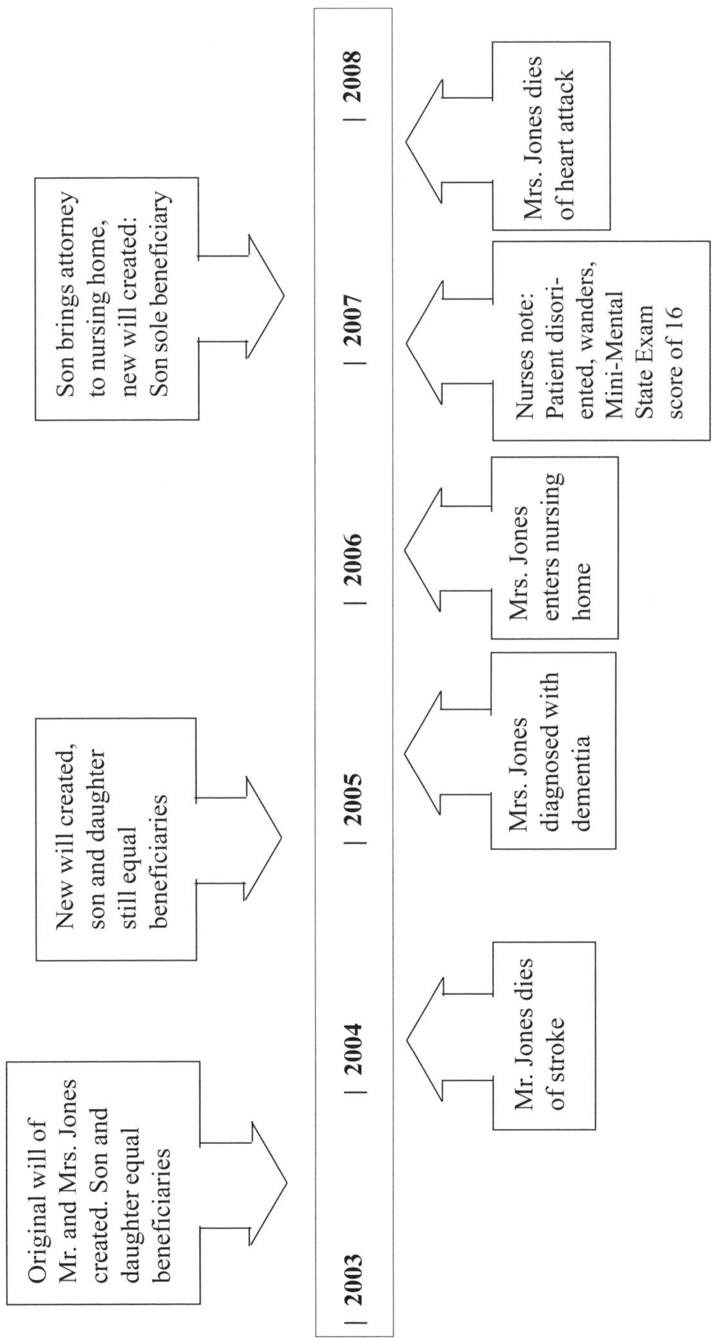

Figure 1. Sample Timeline

testator should be assessed to determine the underlying cause of the observed deficits in order to provide this information to the fact finder. The extent of this assessment will vary depending on circumstances. For example, a testator may be in a nursing home and under the care of a psychiatrist or neurologist who has performed a diagnostic assessment utilizing advanced imaging techniques and clinical evaluation. As a result, there may already be a well-supported diagnosis of a condition such as Alzheimer's disease that readily explains the testator's inability to grasp the process of making a will. In other cases, the evaluator may need to perform diagnostic testing sufficient to explain the observed deficits.

As far as the actual techniques that should be utilized in the assessment, a thorough mental status examination (MSE) should always be performed. This is the foundation of nearly all forensic assessments, and evaluation of testamentary capacity is no exception. A properly administered mental status examination will assist in diagnosis through the systematic collection of data regarding the testator's orientation, memory, affect, presence of a thought disorder, and overall mental state. It can also help to generate hypotheses for further testing.

It is important to note that the term *mental status examination* is used to denote several different types of procedures. On the one hand, there is a wide range of brief instruments that are referred to as mental status examinations that are actually cognitive screeners. The most popular of these is the Mini-Mental State Examination (MMSE) which is often used in hospitals and nursing homes to screen for cognitive status (Shulman & Feinstein, 2003). These instruments have their place in these settings but have limited utility in assessments of testamentary capacity for a number of reasons. The first of these is that although most of them have high specificity, they produce few false positive results; those doing poorly on the MMSE are almost certainly cognitively impaired (Shulman & Feinstein, 2003). But they also have relatively poor sensitivity; that is, they produce a high level of false negative diagnoses; those with cognitive impairments may be scored as not having problems. The second is that they do not provide very much data that are helpful in explaining any functional deficits related to the forensic question under consideration.

It should be mentioned that there are a number of reasonably comprehensive mental status/cognitive screening batteries that fall midway between the very brief MSEs mentioned above and that have utility in certain circumstances. Many of these are described and reviewed in *Quick Cognitive Screening for Clinicians: Mini Mental, Clock-Drawing and Other Brief Tests* by Shulman and Feinstein (2003). Some of these instruments can be used as screening batteries either alone or in combination and may be used when a subject is bedridden, has visual impairments, or in other related circumstances. A number of these mental status batteries are reasonably comprehensive and may be the choice of evaluators when the subject has specific perceptual sensory or motoric impairments that make psychological testing problematic. (Also see the list of semistructured instruments and clinical tools that are included on the CD-Rom accompanying this book.)

It is generally unnecessary to administer the type of highly comprehensive cognitive and neuropsychological battery that one might utilize in a cognitive rehabilitation setting where a very detailed and fine-grained picture of all aspects of the subject's cognitive functioning needs to be described. Again, this is because the standard for testamentary capacity is set low, and it is unlikely that mild cognitive limitation would be sufficient to cause significant functional deficits. Further, it is not uncommon to encounter problematic assessments of testamentary capacity performed by well-trained neuropsychologists who did not completely understand the nature of the forensic issues in these types of cases. When this occurs, one can sometimes observe a tendency to conflate the finding of neuropsychological issues with the presence or absence of testamentary capacity. This basic misunderstanding is seen in other areas of forensic practice; clinicians will sometimes equate the presence of mental retardation with parental incapacity or a psychosis with incapacity to proceed in a criminal case. This error occurs when clinicians confuse what could potentially be a causal aspect of observed incapacity (mental retardation, psychosis) with functional incapacity.

In the real world, some individuals with mental retardation are quite capable of adequate parenting, and most psychotic persons are able to stand trial. Subnormal IQ or schizophrenia could be the underlying cause for observed incapacity in a particular individual, but the diagnosis is not synonymous with an opinion regarding incapacity. Finally, not all aspects of cognitive functioning are likely to have an effect one way or another on an individual's testamentary capacity. Although deficits in reasoning, problem solving, memory, and orientation are likely to be factors underlying testamentary capacity, problems in praxis, nonverbal reasoning, and other areas of mental functioning are less likely to be involved and need not be as extensively assessed.

As with all psychological assessments, the techniques utilized should be designed to address the referral question thoroughly and expeditiously. Test selection is in large part a matter of professional judgment and personal taste. It is not our intention to provide an exhaustive list of tests and techniques that can be used for assessment of testamentary capacity; interested readers are referred to the latest edition of *Evaluating Competencies* by Thomas Grisso (2003). It is an excellent resource for approaching a wide variety of competency assessments; he also provides detailed reviews of many tests designed to assist with such evaluations.

The following description of a suggested methodology for assessment of testamentary capacity is designed to provide a practical starting point for clinicians working in this area of practice.

THE MENTAL STATUS EVALUATION

It is always important to administer a mental status examination, which is the cornerstone of a good forensic evaluation. There are many ways to do this effectively. Some professionals prefer to work from memory and perform the MSE extemporaneously. Others use a checklist or interview driver. Using such checklists has a number of advantages. First, checklists ensure that the clinician will ask all of the questions that may prove relevant to the case. This is useful when writing the report and also when being deposed or giving testimony. Often, opposing counsel will ask many questions about what areas the expert explored in examination of the testator, not so much because they are relevant, but because a succession of answers indicating areas that the expert did not inquire about gives the appearance of an incomplete assessment. When this cross-examination technique is utilized, the clinician can simply refer to the Mental Status Examination Checklist (MSEC) and state exactly what the subject said in response to each question. A number of other semistructured instruments and clinical tools are included on the CD-Rom that accompanies this book.

A second reason for using structured or semistructured MSE forms is that it is clear from years of empirical research that the use of such interviews is a more effective way of eliciting accurate information than free-wheeling clinical examination, as pointed out by Richard Rogers in his excellent book *Handbook of Diagnostic and Structured Interviewing* (Rogers, 2001). Finally, as Rogers made clear in his book, by using structured interview techniques, the interview can become a type of objective instrument. Part of being an expert is pattern recognition as well as attention to details that nonexperts miss. When the evaluator uses a structured interview as part of the assessment of many different individuals, the evaluator becomes able to compare responses across individuals and note differences that may be indicative of particular issues. If the examiner uses a more free-wheeling style of interviewing, he or she may never have the same data set twice, making pattern recognition much more difficult.

There are many excellent mental status forms that are commercially available. One that is particularly useful is the Mental Status Checklist for Adults published by Psychological Assessment Resources (Schinka, 1988). It is comprehensive and works well as an interview driver. In addition, PAR also sells a computer report writer program that allows the psychologist or clerical staff to transfer the subject's answers to the computer, which then outputs a narrative report. The report will need editing to make it flow and match the evaluator's writing style, but despite this it saves a great deal of time. After all, there are only so many ways to say "the subject's speech was normal in quantity and quality and no articulation problems were noted" or "the client was of average height." Other mental status forms are available from other sources. On their website, John Wiley and Sons (Wiley, 2001) has a section called "Theraforms" which provides a variety of mental status, personal history, and clinical interview forms that can be downloaded for a small charge and copied freely by the purchaser.

In administering the mental status interview, it is important to explain to subjects that it is not a test and that if they do not know the answer to a question, they should report if they are approximating or guessing. It is helpful to tell subjects that if the evaluator checks something off and has not asked a question, he or she is simply recording something which was observed and did not require a question, such as the color of their hair or if they wear glasses. Further, they should be told that if they are asked a question such as "Do you hear people talking to you that other people cannot hear?," it is not necessarily because they look like they are hallucinating; rather, everybody is asked the same questions. These explanations can help put the subject at ease. Also, starting with the mental status interview helps subjects to relax in the interview, since they need only to answer yes or no or give brief responses.

THE CLINICAL INTERVIEW

Having completed the mental status interview, the evaluator will move on to the clinical interview. The authors have developed the Semi-Structured Interview for the Assessment of Testamentary Capacity (SSIATC), which is designed to serve as an *aide memoir* for the assessment of testamentary capacity and undue influence. It is included on the CD-Rom accompanying this book and can be reproduced freely. The interview is designed to move from general issues to more specific questions with direct bearing on the testator's capacities with regard to making a will or similar legal document. The interview starts with questions about the subject's personal history, including family of origin, education, and occupational history. Queries regarding important interpersonal relationships are also made. These questions elicit information relevant to testators' understanding of the natural objects of their bounty. The interview then moves on to explore the subject's medical history, including past serious illnesses and injuries, chronic conditions, and current medical status. Subjects' understanding of their treatment and prognosis is also explored.

It should be understood that information not directly related to the execution of a will or trust can still be very important in assisting the court in making decisions about capacity. This is because even when the testator is alive and available for examination, the majority of assessments of testamentary capacity will still be retrospective in nature. The assessment is designed to provide information about the testator's mental state at the time the legal documents were executed, and generally the examination will not take place contemporaneously, although such screenings do occur on occasion, generally when the testator expects that there will be resistance to changes in the will. But in many cases, the person sitting across the table from the examiner will be very different from the individual who signed the will 6 months ago. His or her cognitive and/or emotional deficits may have worsened since that time due to the progression of a disease or new neurological insults. On the other hand, he or she may have been depressed or delirious at the time of the execution of the will, and these symptoms may now have abated. Interviews and testing of the subject allow the psychologist to produce a snapshot of the subject's current cognitive and emotional functioning, but also help to make an informed estimate of the subject's likely level of functioning at the time the will or trust was signed.

It is possible that the subject is now confused about the terms of the will and the reasons for his or her choices at the time, and the examiner may have to make a judgment, based on the nature of the underlying deficits, that it is likely that the subject was or was not equally confused at the time of execution of the will or trust. For example, the fact that the subject is also confused or misinformed about his or her health and educational and occupational history adds weight to the judgment that the subject was in a similar state of confusion 6 months ago.

The clinical interview moves on to explore the subject's current living situation. The subject is questioned about sources of financial support and asked about assets. Questions should start out with open-ended prompts designed to elicit a free narrative, but if subjects have difficulty with this, they can be asked specific questions about their checking and savings accounts, pensions, properties, and indebtedness. These questions are designed to provide information related to the legal issue of the testator's knowledge of the assets that will be distributed in the will.

Subjects are then asked specific questions about the purpose of a will or trust and the changes they have made or contemplate making. Questions include:

- What is a (will, trust, etc.)?
- Who are the immediate members of your family?
- Why do people have them?
- Do you have one?
- Did you have one before the latest one?
- How is the new one different from the last one?
- Why are you making these changes?
- With whom did you discuss these changes?
- Do you have any misgivings about these changes? (Why or why not?)

Testators should be allowed to provide their understanding of these issues, as well as providing their reasons for making changes in their estate planning. The examiner should prompt subjects to provide more information if their answers are limited or sketchy. This is important, because some individuals with cognitive limitations have a tendency to answer with short, rehearsed "set piece" answers that can give the impression of understanding when there is none. Similar types of verbalizations can also be seen in sleep talkers; they relate to an emotionally charged event but have no actual content. Confabulatory answers can also be a problem in these cases. This occurs when an individual with memory loss deals with the absence of a specific memory by creating a narrative of what occurred that can in some cases be convincing, but is actually false. This process is unconscious and is one way in which some impaired individuals deal with gaps in their recollections. These problems underline why some way of corroborating testators' accounts is essential, because otherwise it would be possible to assume that they have capacity when they in fact do not.

*PSYCHOLOGICAL TESTING**

If, after completing the interview, the evaluator believes that the subject has impairments that may be relevant to decisions regarding capacity, the examination moves to the next phase. This involves formal testing to determine the presence or absence of such deficits and their severity if present. This part of the assessment also relates to the causal component of Grisso's (2003) methodology. In this section of the assessment, tests are utilized to measure the subject's general intellectual ability and general cognitive status. It should be noted that some individuals, particularly the elderly, can become fatigued by the interview. When signs of fatigue or frustration appear, it is often best to discontinue the assessment and reschedule for later in the day or for another day.

The assessment can begin with one of the briefer IQ test in order to establish an estimate of the subject's current cognitive capacity. The authors generally do not administer the WAIS-IV (Wechsler, 2008), as the test is time-consuming and can tire an elderly subject. Also, the relatively low standard for testamentary capacity generally makes the use of the full WAIS-IV unnecessary. There are any number of briefer measures that can be utilized which provide reliable, valid measures

* **Note**. Technical information regarding all of the psychometric tests mentioned in this book can be found at the Buros Institute of Mental Measurement website: http://buros.unl.edu/buros/jsp/search.jsp

of current intellectual functioning. These include the Wechsler Abbreviated Scale of Intelligence (WASI; Wechsler, 1999) and the Kaufman Brief Intelligence Test-2 (KBIT-2; A. S. Kaufman & N. L. Kaufman, 2004), which both have good psychometric properties and correlate well with WAIS-IV full scale IQ. One excellent alternative to the WAIS-IV is the Reynolds Intellectual Assessment Scales (RIAS; Reynolds & Kamphaus, 1998). It is more comprehensive than the brief tests mentioned above but is still quicker to administer than the full WAIS. It has optional verbal and nonverbal memory scales that are not utilized in computing the IQ scores but which may be useful when memory problems related to dementia or related conditions are an issue. Finally, the test has no motor component and does not require reading, which can be helpful with subjects who have limitations in those areas. The RIAS also includes a two-scale brief version of itself called the Reynolds Intellectual Screening Test (RIST) which can be useful in certain circumstances. The IQCODE that we have included on the CD-Rom accompanying this book can also be utilized.

Once an IQ test is administered, the examiner should administer tests to assess specific aspects of cognition. As previously stated, it is not generally necessary to administer a comprehensive neuropsychological battery such as the Halstead-Reitan (Reitan & Wolfson, 1993) or the Neuropsychological Assessment Battery (Stern & White, 2003) in these types of assessments. There are many briefer neuropsychological batteries that can be utilized that provide important information regarding reasoning, memory, orientation, language comprehension, and other cognitive domains. The Repeatable Battery for the Assessment of Neuropsychological Status (RBANS; Randolf, 1998) is a relatively brief battery that provides subtests which assess Learning, Story Memory, Figure Copy, Line Orientation, Digit Span, Coding, Picture Naming, Semantic Fluency, List Recall, List Recognition, Story Recall, and Figure Recall. The MicroCog (Powell et al., 2004) is a computer-based neuropsychological battery. It is flexible, and has short (30-minute) and comprehensive (60-minute) forms; the examiner can also pick and choose among the subtests for a customized battery. One caveat regarding the test is that some elderly subjects are unused to using a computer and a mouse and find the test difficult for this reason.

Another test that is useful in this area of forensic assessment is the Dementia Rating Scale-2 (DRS-2; Jurica, Leitten, & Mattis, 2001).

The test allows for brief and comprehensive administration and is designed with a low "floor" so that even very low functioning individuals can be assessed. The DRS-2 has subtests – Attention, Initiation/Perseveration, Construction, Conceptualization, and Memory – and is a good choice for assessments of testamentary capacity and undue influence with elderly subjects.

In performing testing in these types of assessments, it is sometimes helpful to use supplemental tests when particular aspects of cognition are of concern. The Delis-Kaplan Executive Function Scale (D-KEFS; Delis, Kaplan, & Kramer, 2001) is a standardized collection of subtests designed to assess cognitive functions associated with the frontal lobes. The examiner can give as many or as few subtests as is deemed appropriate, and the subject's performance can give important information about reasoning ability. Such results can help explain observed deficits in rational understanding and decision making. Some clinicians prefer to utilize additional memory tests or batteries such as the Wechsler Memory Scales (Wechsler, 1997), the Wide Range Assessment of Memory and Learning - Second Edition (WRAML2; Sheslow & Adams, 2003) or shorter tests such as the Rey Auditory Verbal Learning Test (Schmidt, 1996). Again, it is important to bear in mind that there is always a trade-off between the nature and amount of information gleaned from the results of testing and the wear and tear on the subject.

EMOTIONAL STATUS

Some type of assessment of the subject's emotional state should also be undertaken, because it is always possible that emotional factors, either alone or in combination with organic issues, may be having an impact on the subject's thought processes. One of the authors was once involved in a case involving an elderly woman whose relatives had gone to court to obtain guardianship over her. She had been seen by a psychiatrist who had referred her for neuropsychological assessment. The neuropsychological examination had revealed many areas of cognitive difficulty, including problems with short-term memory, orientation, and constructional abilities. On the basis of this testing, the subject was diagnosed with moderate dementia, most probably of the Alzheimer's type. The woman's lawyer contacted the author about the possibility of providing a second opinion. When these types of referrals occur, it is often helpful to suggest that the examination be postponed until the information from the previous examination is reviewed. This allows a determination as to whether further input is likely to be helpful.

In this case, when the neuropsychological report was reviewed, it was seen that in addition to clinically depressed scores on a number of tests, the subject had also obtained a clinically elevated score on the Beck Depression Inventory (Beck, Steer, & Brown, 1996). A review of the history section of the report revealed that the subject had suffered an injury earlier in the year and that her general condition had deteriorated around that time. This raised the possibility that, rather than being demented, the subject might actually be suffering from pseudodementia. The subject's lawyer was contacted and it was suggested that she be seen by a geropsychiatrist to determine if this was the case prior to pursuing further assessment. The psychiatrist confirmed the presence of pseudodementia, treated the subject with an antidepressant, and it was reported that she was doing much better. When a forensic assessment which included a clinical interview, record review, mental status examination, the RBANS (Randolf, 1998), and selected subtests of the D-KEFS (Delis et al., 2001) was performed, all scores were normal, and it was clear that the subject was not demented. Although this case dealt with guardianship rather than testamentary capacity, it points out the necessity for assessing the subject's emotional state and developing appropriate hypotheses.

As with cognitive assessment, in assessing the subject's emotional state, the clinician must strike a balance between employing techniques that help answer the diagnostic question without unduly tiring the subject. It is probably best to avoid unidimensional scale tests in favor of multiscale instruments such as the MMPI-2 (Butcher et al., 1989), Personality Assessment Inventory (PAI; Morey, 1991), Basic Personality Inventory (Jackson, 1988), and Coolidge Assessment Battery (Coolidge, 1999). These instruments cover more diagnostic possibilities than the unidimensional scales. At the same time, the evaluator should be cognizant that tests such as the MMPI-2 may be too long for many subjects in these types of assessments. Depending on the situation, the short form of the MMPI-2 could be utilized as well as the new MMPI-2-RF (Ben Porath, & Tellegen, 2008); this approach is justified given the nature of the referral question and the legal standards in these types of cases. Also, the new MMPI-2-RF (Ben Porath & Tellegen, 2008) is shorter than the MMPI-2 (Butcher et al., 1989); it shows great promise as a next generation personality test and may be used in some circumstances. The fact that the MMPI-2-RF will read itself to the subject using the computer's speakers is also very helpful with subjects with compromised vision or other reading problems.

CONTEXTUAL ISSUES

Once the questions raised by the causal component of the five-step model (Grisso, 2003) have been addressed, the evaluator can turn to the interactive issues. One of the contextual variables raised in assessments of testamentary capacity is the extent of the testator's estate and complexity of his or her finances. It would be easier to have a general grasp of the extent of one's property and finances when the estate consists of a house, car, and pension than if the estate consists of a large stock portfolio, multiple bank accounts, several properties, and a majority interest in a working corporation. In the same way, a testator who has only married once and has two living children will have an easier time recognizing the natural objects of his or her bounty than a person who has divorced twice and remarried three times, with children from two of the marriages. These types of contextual issues should be considered in terms of how they relate to the testator's mental capacities. In cases involving deceased testators, this component could be assessed retrospectively, assuming sufficient documentation exists to allow an opinion to be formulated with a reasonable degree of certainty.

THE ULTIMATE ISSUE/CONCLUSARY ASPECT AND REMEDIATION

There is ongoing controversy regarding whether mental health professionals should opine regarding the ultimate issue. However, it has been our experience that attorneys and, more importantly, the courts expect to hear the professional's opinion about whether the testator possessed testamentary capacity or not. We have found that the best way to express such an opinion in reports is to state it as follows: "While decisions regarding the ultimate issue rest with the court, it is my opinion that the testator did/did not possess testamentary capacity at the time of his/her revision of the will."

Finally, there may be cases in which steps may be taken that may render a testator who currently lacks testamentary capacity capable of making or changing a will. For example, it may be the case that an elderly testator thought to be primarily demented may actually be psychotically depressed. In such a case, a recommendation could be made for psychiatric intervention and reexamination at a future date. Obviously, this component would not apply to deceased testators.

ASSESSMENT OF UNDUE INFLUENCE

The assessment of undue influence involves all of the components of the evaluation of testamentary capacity, with a number of added considerations. It should be noted that if there is a lack of testamentary capacity, there cannot be a finding of undue influence, because there would be no rational intent of the testator to influence.

In cases involving living testators, the evaluator should interview them carefully regarding the reasons for the choices they have made in writing or modifying their will. Subjects should also be questioned regarding their day-to-day life in order to elicit data that would shed light on the extent to which they did or did not have a confidential relationship with the beneficiary of the will. Additionally, information should be elicited about who controls the subject's finances and the extent to which the beneficiary controlled access to and communication with others. Generally, there should be an investigation of the extent to which the testator was dependant on the beneficiary.

The reasons for the testator's deviation from traditional patterns of wealth dispersion should be explored, as well as the reason for any change from previous expressed desires in this regard. An evaluation similar to that described in the section on testamentary capacity should be performed to determine if testators suffered from a mental condition which had the potential to render them more susceptible to undue influence. This information should be integrated with information regarding the aforementioned seven indicia noted by Spar and Garb (1992).

In cases involving a deceased testator, the presence or absence of these indicia should be described, and a retrospective analysis of the testator's mental state should be performed to the extent possible in the same manner as would be done in retrospective assessments of testamentary capacity.

ASSESSMENT AT THE TIME THE WILL IS EXECUTED

Many of the problems that lead to legal challenges of wills could be avoided if testators were assessed at the time they actually made their will. This would be particularly helpful if there is reason to suspect that a relative or other party is likely to contest a will on the grounds of undue influence or incapacity. This practice has become more common among lawyers who engage in probate law. In such evaluations, videotaping is recommended to preserve a record which can be brought into court. Such examinations generally include a mental status examination, a clinical interview which addresses all of the components of testamentary capacity, and the administration of screening tests such as the Mini-Mental State Examination (MMSE) to address the causal component of testamentary capacity (Shulman & Feinstein, 2003).

TESTIMONY IN TESTAMENTARY CAPACITY AND UNDUE INFLUENCE CASES

Although some percentage of cases involving testamentary capacity and undue influence settle before they reach probate court, the evaluator in these cases may be called to testify regarding his or her conclusions. In such cases it is important to present conclusions in a manner that will assist the fact finder and minimize the chances that testimony will be misinterpreted. The following information, presented in the appropriate sequence, will help accomplish these goals.

1. A general description of the testator's general functional state should be presented. This information should be presented in plain English and use examples drawn from the records in the case, the results of testing (whether administered by the expert or drawn from the record), and the implications of such results and face-to-face interviews in the case of living subjects. If there is a definitive diagnosis with clear implications for the case, it should be presented and explained.
2. The expert should take pains to explain that the presence or absence of a particular condition such as dementia is not the same as a finding of incapacity. This is especially important if the testator was demented or psychotic at the time of the creation or modification of the will, but the expert believes that capacity

was present, due to evidence of a lucid interval or sufficient residual mental faculties.

3. The expert should present his or her opinion on the ultimate issue along with a concise summary of the reasons for reaching these conclusions.

In conclusion, it has been our experience in cases of testamentary capacity and undue influence that if the five-step model (Grisso, 2003) is carefully utilized and pains are taken to testify in the manner outlined above, the expert witness will be able to effectively assist the court in making determinations in these matters.

APPENDIX

Case Studies

Case Studies*

Case Study 1: Testamentary Capacity – Deceased Testator

The following case involves the testamentary capacity of a testator who was deceased at the time of my assessment. In this case, I (Dr. Mart) summarized my findings in a letter to the attorney who had retained me and did not complete a formal psychological report. This occurred for several reasons. First, the summary was needed to serve as my expert disclosure letter; when expert witnesses are going to be utilized in a case (probate or other), opposing counsel must be given notice about the use of the expert and the matters on which he or she will testify. At that point, opposing counsel can decide whether or not to proceed with a deposition of the expert. In this case, the matter was settled out of court prior to my testifying or being deposed, so there was no need to do further work on the case. I have included this case study to provide information about how to proceed in the case of a deceased testator.

It should be noted that the example given here was a fairly uncomplicated case in which there was a great deal of clear-cut evidence both from medical records and from witnesses. In other situations, retrospective analysis of a testator's state of mind at the time a will or trust was executed can be far more ambiguous, and greater efforts may have to be made to gather evidence from a wide range of sources. Additional sources of information may include multiple interviews with individuals who interacted with the testator in many different roles. These can include home health care aides; physical, occupational, and respiratory therapists; nursing home staff (both medical and administrative); friends; clergy; and trades persons. In some cases, financial records can be reviewed to determine the extent to which the individual was managing his or her own financial affairs in the months leading up to the signing of the document in question. Differential effects of medications, bereavement, or acute or chronic psychiatric problems may have to be factored into the analysis. From both practical and ethical standpoints, the retrospective analyses of mental states such

*Names and identifying characteristics in all case examples have been changed to protect confidentiality.

as testamentary capacity and undue influence must be sufficiently comprehensive to provide support for the conclusions reached by experts in their final reports.

Further, as previously noted, there is some disagreement in the forensic mental health field as to whether experts should give opinions about the ultimate issue, particularly with regard to issues such as testamentary capacity and undue influence when the testator is deceased. Those opposed to providing such an opinion point out that concepts such as capacity and undue influence are legal rather than psychological constructs and therefore, an expert giving such an opinion represents an unjustified intrusion into the province of the court. Those who support experts giving such opinions note that judges and juries are empowered to give such opinions as much or as little weight as they choose based on the foundation for the opinion laid by the expert testimony.

This is a matter that each expert must resolve for himself or herself. In my experience, judges and juries almost always want to know my opinion regarding the ultimate issue, whether the case involves mental state at time of offense, competence to stand trial, child custody and visitation, testamentary capacity, or undue influence. My solution is to remind the judge or jury in my testimony and reports that my opinion on the ultimate issue is only one aspect of my work on a particular case prior to actually rendering my opinion.

In this case, Mr. Jones was an elderly white male who lived in a small town in Vermont. Because he lived very frugally and invested successfully in mutual funds that appreciated over the years, he left a substantial estate at the time of his death. He was survived by his mother, who was nearly 95 years old at the time her son died. He had not married and had no children. To summarize my assessment techniques, I wrote the following to the attorney who had retained my services:

> I am writing to provide you with my preliminary report regarding Richard A. Jones. In preparation for this report I have reviewed the medical records you provided. In addition, I have conducted interviews of Herbert Frost, Robert LeClerc, and Casey Dawson. I will be reviewing other information as it becomes available.

In this case there was little information about Mr. Jones prior to his final illness. However, in his later years, he and Herbert Frost and Robert LeClerc (two friends who were also retired) spent nearly every day sitting around Mr. Jones's woodworking shop, discussing the events of the day and reminiscing. These two individuals were good sources of data because they did not have an interest in the will and had also seen Mr. Jones before he became ill and at the time the new will was executed. Casey Dawson was the niece of Mr. Jones's long-time female companion, and she cared for him from the time he left the hospital until he died. The medical file revealed the following information:

> To summarize, Mr. Jones was an individual who did not obtain medical care from the 1980s until his admission to the University of Vermont Hospital in late July of 2006. At that time he was diagnosed with malignant hypertension, cerebrovascular accident and a neoplasm of unknown primary origin. At the time of his hospitalization his cancer had metastasized widely through his body, and lesions were found in the frontal, parietal, and temporal lobes of his brain. Although initially he was minimally responsive, his neurological state over his hospitalization improved to the point where he was described as verbal and able to follow commands. However, it was also noted that he evidenced confusion and confabulation.

As I mentioned in an earlier chapter, medical records that are contemporaneous or near contemporaneous with the execution of a questionable will are often a rich source of data regarding the testator's state of mind at the time of the will's execution. This can be particularly true of nursing home records, because they are required to do a number of different types of assessments by the government in order to be eligible for funding. After spending time in the hospital, Mr. Jones's doctors decided that his case was terminal and that palliative care was most appropriate. He was transferred to a nursing home that had a hospice wing. Further examination of the medical records from this admission provided the following data:

> Mr. Jones was transferred to River View Nursing Home on 8/8/06. He was administered the Mini-Mental Exam on 8/13/06. At that time, Mr. Jones did not know the year, season, date, day, or month. He was oriented to place and was able to respond correctly to questions about his location at that time including country, state, county, town, and the name of his facility. He was unable to perform serial sevens or

> spell "world" backward. He was unable to recall three words which he had been taught several minutes earlier. He obtained a score of 15 on the examination which is consistent with moderately severe dementia. Notes on the protocol state "resident staring and no response to many questions." In response to be asked to write a sentence and copy a simple design, "resident put paper down and would not attempt to write or draw even with encouragement." Mr. Jones was also administered the Clock Drawing Task, which is a widely used procedure for measuring cognitive deficits. The Clock Drawing Task measures a wide range of intellectual and perceptual skills including comprehension, planning, visual spatial abilities, abstract thinking, and concentration. In the version of the test given to Mr. Jones on 8/13/06, he was asked to draw the face of the clock, put the numbers in the correct positions, and then draw in the hands at 10 minutes after 11. There are a number of scoring systems for this test, but Mr. Jones's drawing was clearly highly deficient. He appears to have made two attempts to draw the clock face: the first has the numeral 1 where the 12 should be, ends with 10 where 11 should be, and has no hands. His second attempt has the numeral 20 where the 12 should be and includes the numerals 13 through 19, again with no hands included. This performance is indicative of disorientation and problems with memory, planning, and reasoning. The medical data available through 8/13/06 clearly points to Mr. Jones being demented, with moderate levels of cognitive impairment present at that time.

Mr. Jones's mother and Casey Dawson became dissatisfied with the care he was receiving at the hospice and decided to move him to Ms. Dawson's home to care for him. Around this time, a local lawyer heard that Mr. Jones was ill and called him to see if he wanted to discuss his estate planning, to which he agreed. On 8/17/06 a meeting with the attorney and a business associate of the attorney took place, and several days later the attorney and his associate came back to see Mr. Jones with a 35-page document for him to sign. Mr. Frost, Mr. LeClerc, and Ms. Dawson were present for the signing.

> Attorney Lamb and Mr. Paulson returned on 8/21/06 to have the estate plan executed. As you are aware, there has been testimony in deposition that Mr. Jones did not ask any questions at either the meeting of the 17th or the 21st. There is also testimony that the documents were not read to Mr. Jones or explained to him. Additionally, witnesses stated that no attempt was made by Attorney Lamb to assess whether Mr. Jones knew what the documents were, understood the extent of

> his assets, or could name the individuals who were the natural objects of his bounty. Mr. Jones passed away on 9/7/2006.

When the documents were examined by the attorney who retained me, it was discovered that contrary to Mr. Jones's lifelong wish that his money and property be distributed to his mother and Ms. Dawson, they were essentially cut out of the will. The new will provided that most of the estate would go to Mr. Paulson, who had very little contact with Mr. Jones prior to his illness and who had never been mentioned in any prior wills. My discussions with witnesses to the signing revealed that Mr. Jones sat mutely before the document at the will signing, seemed confused and disoriented, asked and answered no questions, and had to be prompted several times over a 20-minute period to sign the will. He did turn the pages, but did not appear to read anything. Based on all of the information I had collected, I concluded:

> Based on my review of the available documentation and my interviews with individuals who know Mr. Jones and were witnesses to some of the events associated with the signing of these estate planning documents, it is my opinion that Mr. Jones had significant and severe cognitive deficits at that time. These deficits included problems with memory, orientation, attention, concentration, and reasoning, and were associated with the lesions in his brain. His frontal lobes, which control executive function (planning, reasoning, task initiation, abstraction), were particularly compromised. Based on all the information available, it is my opinion that Mr. Jones lacked testamentary capacity at the time 8/21/06 estate planning documents were executed.

It should be noted that there was much more information available in this situation than is usually the case. Mr. Jones had been screened for cognitive deficits around the time the new will was signed, and he was observed by individuals who knew him well before and after he was diagnosed with brain cancer. Having this data made it much easier to draw conclusions about his capacity at the time of his execution of the disputed will. In cases where the data are not so clear cut, the psychologist will either have to limit the scope of his or her conclusions or refrain from speculating where the data do not support such conclusions to a reasonable degree of certainty. It should be kept in mind that it is an affirmative ethical obligation to reveal limitations imposed by sparse data to the court.

Case Study 2:
Testamentary Capacity – Living Testator

This case involved a living testator who was 85 years old at the time I evaluated him. I had been contacted by his attorney who explained the basis of the case. Mr. Smith had owned a garage that had been profitable and, being a frugal man, had a substantial estate. According to the attorney, as Mr. Smith had become older and less vigorous, he had allowed his eldest son from his first marriage to work with him in the garage and gradually allowed him to take over more and more day-to-day running of the establishment. Eventually, Mr. Smith let his son take over his financial affairs, and his only real role was to sign the papers that his son placed before him. Mr. Smith and his wife became concerned in the summer of 2007 when his son began to liquidate some of their property without consulting them. When they confronted the son with their objections, he presented them documents signed by Mr. Smith that showed that he transferred much of their property to the son's control. In addition, Mr. Smith became aware that he had signed a revised will in 2006 that made his son, rather than his wife, the main beneficiary of his estate. It was at this point that Mr. and Mrs. Smith consulted their lawyer and found that Mr. Smith had unknowingly signed a new will that would make his son the sole heir to his estate, and which excluded Mrs. Smith almost completely. Mr. Smith's lawyer checked into the matter further and found that Mr. Smith had been diagnosed with a neurological condition some years previous to the time the documents were signed. It was for this reason that he questioned Mr. Smith's testamentary capacity and requested that I perform a psychological evaluation.

Over the years I have developed a format for forensic reports that I find meets my needs and the needs of counsel. I will describe the process I went through in evaluating Mr. Smith following the structure of my report. The reader will probably have his or her own way of structuring assessments and reports; this is to a large extent a matter of experience and personal preference. At the same time, I believe an effective forensic report should accomplish several tasks.

1. It should explain what you did in a clear, concise manner that is understandable by nonpsychologists.

2. It should allow the reader to understand how you arrived at your conclusions; there should be a logical nexus between your data and your conclusion. Just as in your high school math classes, you should "show your work."
3. It should proceed in a logical manner that allows the reader to understand why you did what you did in the assessment so that they can make independent decisions about the validity of your conclusions.

I begin my reports with a "reason for referral" section that sets up the purpose of the assessment and explains what I was trying to determine. In this case, I stated the following:

> Mr. Smith was referred by his attorney for psychological evaluation. Mr. Smith is currently involved in a court case which involves his will as well as issues related to his past management of his financial affairs. The evaluation was requested to provide the court with information about his general cognitive and functional capacity, his testamentary capacity, and his ability to give accurate and reliable responses in deposition and testimony.

This section is also an excellent place to insert information about any limitations on your data that have the potential to affect your conclusions, and also to make any necessary statements regarding the scope of your assessment. For example, if the testator is deceased at the time of your assessment, you could include a statement such as this:

> Mr. Jones was deceased at the time this evaluation was requested. For this reason, it was not possible to conduct a personal interview as a part of this assessment. The conclusions in this report were drawn from a careful examination of Mr. Jones's medical records, interviews with his treating physicians, and other collateral data sources as detailed in the body of this report.

I follow this section with a list of the methods I used in the assessment titled "Evaluation Techniques." In this case, I used the following methods:

- Record Review
- Clinical Interview

- Mental Status Checklist for Adults
- Mini-Mental State Examination
- Repeatable Battery for the Assessment of Neuropsychological Status-Form A

I will explain my choice of techniques in this case and what they did or did not show as I come to each one.

My next section in nearly all of my reports is a section that lays out the information I elicited from the records I was able to review. In this case, a discovery packet had been put together by both lawyers, so I had complete medical records for the period surrounding the events in the case. The following is my description of the parts of the medical records that I felt had a direct bearing on the issues in the case:

> As part of this assessment, I reviewed medical records provided to me by Mr. Smith's attorney. The bulk of these records are related to a number of medical conditions, including an eye injury, gallbladder surgery, and carotid stenosis, and had no direct bearing on my assessment. However, he was seen by Dr. Mary Lindner in 2003 for complaints of giddiness and balance problems. He received a CT scan of his brain on 8/8/03. The radiological report notes that Mr. Smith exhibited "Relative enlargement of the 3rd ventricle and lateral ventricle with sparing of the 4th ventricle. Differential considerations include normal pressure hydrocephalus or periventricular white matter tissue loss. MRI of the brain should be considered for further evaluation." A report dated 10/13/03 by Dr. Lindner noted continued problems with balance. At the time of this examination he scored 28 out of 30 on the Mini-Mental State Examination, which falls in the normal range. Dr. Lindner noted that the results of the previously mentioned CT scan made her suspicious that he might be suffering from central atrophy of the brain. I spoke to his wife, Dorothy Smith, and she told me that Mr. Smith's doctors now feel that he had some type of stroke in 2002 or 2003 which was the underlying cause of his symptoms. Her account was confirmed in records from his current PCP received after this conversation.

It was important to include this information because it provides evidence that some type of neurological problem was evident as early as 2003. Although his MMSE score was in the normal range at that time, it must be understood that the MMSE has high specificity but low sensitivity (Shulman & Feinstein, 2003). This means that below-average scores are generally indicative of cognitive deficits, average scores are not necessarily evidence that cognitive problems are absent, and the test has a high false negative rate. Further, even if Mr. Smith was not immediately demonstrating cognitive limitations in 2003, it is likely that the onset of his symptoms marked the beginning of a degenerative process.

My next step was to administer a mental status examination to Mr. Smith. This section of the report read as follows:

> As part of this evaluation I administered the Mental Status Checklist for Adults to Mr. Smith. Mr. Smith is an elderly African American male whose appearance is consistent with his chronological age. He is above average in height and of average build. His eyes are brown and his hair is white. Mr. Smith was casually dressed and his hygiene was good. He uses a cane when walking and has an eye patch that covers his injured eye. He has a wide-based gait. At the time of the interview Mr. Smith's motor behavior was normal. He was alert and evidenced no distress during the interview. His facial expression was normal and responsive and his eye contact was appropriately focused. Mr. Smith's speech was normal in both quantity and quality. His mood was calm and cheerful and his affect was appropriate to the content of our discussion. He reports no symptoms of depression or anxiety. Mr. Smith's thought processes were logical and coherent and he gave no evidence of delusional thinking. He denied any compulsions or obsessions and gave no indications of phobic anxiety. Mr. Smith denied any history of hallucinations or recent disturbances of consciousness. He appeared to be of at least average intelligence and his fund of information was consistent with his background. There were no obvious deficits in abstract reasoning ability. Mr. Smith reported some difficulties with his memory.
>
> Mr. Smith told me that he is currently under medical care but could not recall which medications he is taking or why he takes them. He told me that he smoked when he was in the Navy but quit smoking after his service. He reported that he drinks one beer per day and denied any history of alcohol or drug abuse. Mr. Smith does not believe that he has had any recent major change in his weight, and told me that his appetite is good. He reports decreased hours of sleep. As regards legal difficulties, he told me that he has a problem with his eldest son and that he has taken his money and property. He denied

> any other legal problems. Mr. Smith told me that he had no history of violent acts toward himself or anyone else. He reports that he is retired and that his previous occupation was that of truck driver. He is a high school graduate. He is in his second marriage and lives with his spouse. He has four adult children, all from his first marriage.

Of note in this section of the report is the fact that Mr. Smith could not recall his medications, which he takes daily, and knew very little about his medical condition. He also reported some memory problems. He was accurate in his recollection that he had four children.

My next step was to perform a clinical interview with Mr. Smith. This stage of the assessment allows me to obtain background on the subject and also ask specific questions about his understanding of his situation. Also, the clinical interview portion of the assessment is where I ask specific questions associated with testamentary capacity. I find that the more relaxed format of the clinical interview allows the subject to tell his story in his own way and also lets me follow up and explore aspects of his narrative in more detail. Mr. Smith told me the following:

> I asked him why he thought his lawyer wanted him to be evaluated. He told me that his eldest son had been "light-fingered with my money." I asked him to explain, and he told me that sometime in the past this son had come to his office and told Mr. Smith that he had lost his job and wanted to work with him. Mr. Smith told me that his son had asked for $400 per week and that he offered him $250, and that this son had taken everything he had. It should be noted that Mr. Smith repeated this statement by way of explanation of his current difficulties in almost the same words on a number of occasions during my evaluation.
>
> I asked him when this had occurred, and he told me that he did not know but thought it might have been 20 years ago. Mr. Smith told me that he had had an automotive garage and that it was his main source of financial support. I asked Mr. Smith what specifically his son had taken from him, and he told me that he had taken the garage which was worth $500,000, and that his son had obtained possession of this piece of property. He also told me that his son had bought a company car for himself without his knowledge. Mr. Smith told me that it was not until his third son became involved that he discovered what had happened.

I asked Mr. Smith how his attorney could help him in his current situation. He told me that his eldest son could not be put in jail because "he had me sign a piece of paper," and that after a while he had signed everything away. I asked him how much money he thought he had lost, and he told me he believed that it was $2,000,000. I asked him whether any other property was involved, and he told me that there was only the garage and that he wanted to get it back. Mr. Smith told me he thinks that the cash he believes his son took from him is gone. I asked him where the case stands at the present time, and he told me that he had had one trial previously and was going to have another in October. Mr. Smith also mentioned that his second son was the one who put his eye out. When I questioned him about this, he told me that it was an accident, but said that his son should not have been in the garage in the first place. He told me that his second son had coupled a hose together improperly and that when Mr. Smith attempted to use it, it flew apart and put his eye out. He repeated this story several times in the course of our interview.

I questioned Mr. Smith about his understanding of wills in general and of his own specifically. He told me that he wrote his youngest son out of his will and that his second son will receive one dollar. I asked him what his will had been like prior to his changing it, and he told me he did not know. He also told me that he did not know whether his sons had been in the will prior to the changes that were made. I asked him where he wanted his money to go now, and he told me that he wanted his money to go to his third son because "he is the honest one." I questioned Mr. Smith about his relationship with his sons, and he told me that he does not see them or speak to any but his third son. He mentioned several times that his youngest son was "dumber than a box of hammers." I asked him when he had made the most recent changes to his will, and he could not tell me. Mr. Smith told me that his third son does not need his money but that he has a daughter and he would like his money to eventually go to his granddaughter. I asked Mr. Smith how many grandchildren he has, and he told me that he has eight, but repeated that all of his money would go to his third son. I asked him what he would receive, and he indicated that his garage was the extent of his assets. Mr. Smith told me that the purpose of a will is to make sure a person's property goes to the proper recipients. Mr. Smith mentioned that he has not yet been able to get his garage back, but that his lawyer is working on it.

> I interviewed Mr. Smith again on 11/14/07, when I returned to his residence to perform more testing. On this occasion he told me that he was working with his attorney because his eldest son "needs to be straightened out," and that he took his money. I asked him how he had obtained the money, and he told me that he had asked for a job, had him sign papers, and taken over "the whole works." He recalled that he has a will, but he thought it was a "living will," and he said that he wanted his money to go to his third son. He made it clear that he does not want his money to go to his eldest son because he is a "lying thief."

It became clear in this section of the evaluation that Mr. Smith was having more difficulty with memory and general appreciation of his situation than initially met the eye. Particularly noticeable was his tendency to perseverate on certain phrases to explain his situation, when it was clear that he had little understanding of what had occurred with his money and his son. These near-confabulatory types of responses are often used by subjects with memory difficulties in an attempt to cover gaps in their recall.

I readministered the Mini-Mental State Examination (MMSE) in order to provide a comparison to his 2003 results. He achieved a score of 27, which was normal for his age and education level and also commensurate with his 2003 administration. My next step was to administer the Repeatable Battery for the Assessment of Neuropsychological Status (RBANS; Randolph, 1998). The RBANS is a brief neuropsychological battery that is designed to detect deficits in a number of areas of cognitive function. I chose this test over a more comprehensive battery for a number of reasons. The first of these is that many elderly subjects in these types of cases have difficulty tolerating longer neuropsychological batteries. Further, because the standard for testamentary capacity is so low, there is generally no need for a neuropsychological testing designed to pick up very subtle deficits. Mild cognitive deficits are not likely enough to render a testator incompetent. What I generally need is a brief neuropsychological battery that is more sensitive than the MMSE but does not require 4 hours to administer. The RBANS is well suited for this purpose.

Mr. Smith's scores on the RBANS were as follows:

Domain	**Index Score**	**Classification**
Immediate Memory	73	Borderline
Visuospatial/ Constructional	81	Low Average
Language	86	Low Average
Attention	82	Low Average
Delayed Memory	48	Extremely Low
Total Score Index	67	Extremely Low

I wrote the following interpretation of his performance in my report:

> Mr. Smith's Total Scale Index Score of 67 places overall level of performance on the RBANS in the Extremely Low range.
>
> Mr. Smith's pattern of performance on the RBANS subtests indicates that he has significant difficulties in immediate memory and delayed memory. His borderline score on the Immediate Memory subtests indicates that he has difficulty remembering information immediately after it is presented. The extremely low score on the Delayed Memory scale indicates that he has severe difficulties with anterograde memory and that there is a rapid decay of information presented to him. His language skills, sustained attention and visuospatial/constructional skills, while below average, are areas of relative strength for him.

I provide my analysis of the case in the Summary and Results section of the report. In this case, I wrote the following:

> The results of this evaluation indicate that Mr. Smith is an individual who has difficulty with memory above and beyond what might be expected in an individual of his age. Because his language skills are for the most part preserved, he can give the initial impression that he has a greater command of the facts of the situation than is actually the case. His memory problems are clearly demonstrated, both in the results of neuropsychological testing and in his presentation during several interviews. Mr. Smith attempts to cover his deficits and confusion through the use of "set piece" stories that he repeats when questioned about certain matters. This can be seen in his near rote repetition of his accounts of certain events, such as the accident that led to the loss of his eye and the events surrounding his current court

case. When he is questioned more closely and in greater detail, it becomes clear that he does not have a good grasp of the specifics of his current situation. There is also evidence that these memory deficits are generalized. For example, he could tell me very little about his medical conditions and had no idea what medications he takes.

With regard to testamentary capacity, Mr. Smith made it clear that he feels defrauded by his eldest son and wishes his estate to be given to his third son when he passes away. There are some indications that he is resentful towards his eldest son and does not want him to inherit from his estate, but he was unable to give me any reason why he feels this way. In addition, he made no mention of his current wife in relation to his will at all. Also, I was struck by the manner in which Mr. Smith repeats certain stories almost verbatim about the events leading up to the current legal problems. Given the results of neuropsychological testing, it is my feeling that these stories are artifacts of memory. By this, I mean that these are short stories that Mr. Smith tells about circumstances, and which he has repeated often but about which he has little real understanding. This can be demonstrated by asking him to expand on his answers and provide details, which he can almost never do.

Mr. Smith's condition appears to be progressive. It is unlikely that it will improve; it will, in all probability, deteriorate. It is more likely than not that the onset of Mr. Smith's condition began as far back as a decade ago and simply went undetected and undiagnosed by the medical professionals as it progressed. Family members, however, such as his wife, Dorothy, appear to have been aware of Mr. Smith's diminishing capacity as far back as 1998/1999, when she discussed with one of Mr. Smith's doctors the possibility that Mr. Smith may have had a "mini-stroke" or a "series of mini-strokes." For the most part, however, the full significance of Mr. Smith's condition appears to have been unrecognized by those close to Mr. Smith, as others simply compensated for his condition by doing for Mr. Smith that which he could no longer do for himself. As the years passed, Mr. Smith's condition probably continued to deteriorate, with Mr. Smith retaining enough of his ability to communicate to make it difficult for others to grasp how significantly his mental abilities were actually impaired.

As a consequence, I do not believe that Mr. Smith currently has the requisite cognitive abilities to be considered to have testamentary capacity. It is my further opinion that it is more likely than not that Mr. Smith was, at least, somewhat enfeebled in 2000 (i.e., at the time

> of the alleged gift transfer of the shares in his company). It is a distinct possibility that he was not capable of grasping the effect that a gift of his stock in his body shop would have on his future financial security and on the financial security of anyone dependent upon him.
>
> As far as Mr. Smith's ability to provide accurate testimony in deposition, I believe that the problems I mentioned regarding immediate and delayed memory described above would make it very difficult for him to cope with the demands of such a proceeding. In my experience, depositions require accurate answers to questions regarding who, what, why, and where, and I do not believe that Mr. Smith has the present ability to respond to such questions accurately. In addition, he would have great difficulty dealing with any type of hypothetical question, and would also become easily confused, and this increases the likelihood of his giving inaccurate answers.

In this summary, I attempt to bring together the data drawn from the different sources of information I utilized for this assessment, which were record review, structured and unstructured interviews, and psychological testing. In such assessments, if the information drawn from different sources is congruent, the psychologist can be reasonably confident about his or her conclusions. If they are contradictory, further data will be required to attempt to explain these contradictory observations and results.

I have also attempted to address each of Grisso's (2003) competence criteria in this diction of the report. In this case, I did note that Mr. Smith had specific functional deficits with regard to his understanding of the testamentary process. He was confused about his assets, what had happened to them, and his current situation. The causal explanation for these observed deficits was his deteriorating cognitive status most likely related to cerebral atrophy and vascular events. Contextual factors included the likely need for Mr. Smith to be deposed, which required cognitive functioning beyond his abilities. My conclusion was that Mr. Smith lacked testamentary capacity, both at the time he made his new will and at the time I assessed him. Finally, because of the progressive nature of the medical condition responsible for his cognitive deterioration, I concluded that his condition could not be remediated to the point where he would have testamentary capacity.

Case Study 3:
Testamentary Capacity and
Undue Influence Assessment – Deceased Testator

This case involved an elderly man who never married, and lived in a house he shared with a male relative. His extended family lived nearby, and he had frequent contact with his adult nieces and nephews. The testator had lived with one of his adult nephews and in several revisions of his will, he had indicated that his estate should be inherited by this nephew in the first instance. However, if this nephew died before the testator, the estate was to be equally shared with his great nieces and nephews. The nephew with whom the testator resided died unexpectedly and Mr. Cohen moved in with another nephew and the nephew's wife. After this move, the testator made a revised will which now left his entire estate to the nephew with whom he now resided, who was also executor of the will. The remaining adult nieces and nephews challenged the will in probate court. In this case I will let the report to the attorney who retained my services speak for itself.

Dear Attorney Johnston:

I am writing to give you my preliminary report regarding my review and conclusions regarding the case of Samuel T. Cohen. Specifically, you asked me to review available records and provide information regarding my opinions as to whether Mr. Cohen had testamentary capacity at the time he prepared his will or whether there were indications that undue influence was a factor in the production of the will. In preparing this report I reviewed the following documents:

1) Motion to Re-Examine Probate Will 10/26/06
2) Last Will and Testament of Samuel T. Cohen 7/8/03
3) Letter from Silas Little, Esq., to Thomas J. Krinos, Esq. 11/30/06 (with attached copy of Last Will and Testament of Samuel T. Cohen Dated 7/8/03 and Unsigned Copy of Last Will and Testament of Samuel T. Cohen Dated 10/1/02)
4) Letter from Elizabeth Johnston with attached Decision (*In Re: Estate of Frederick W. Whitmore*)

5) Medical Records of Gary M. Johnson, M.D., regarding Samuel Cohen
6) Letters from:
   a. John and Marjorie Johnson
   b. Karen Krantz
   c. Shirley and Joseph Long
   d. Eldon Michaels
   e. Dariel Peterson
   f. Josephine and Francisco Perez
   g. Mary Curtis, LNA
7) Petitioner's First Set of Interrogatories and Request for Production of Documents to Be Answered by J.K., Executor
8) Deposition of J.K. (5/31/07)
9) Medical Records Summary
10) Medical Records of Samuel Cohen
    a. Southfield Family Practice
    b. Cardiology Associates of Ashland County
    c. Green Mountain Internists
    d. Samuel Gold, M.D.
    e. Green Mountain Community Hospital
    f. Long Pond Healthcare
    g. Medical Records of Gary M. Johnson, M.D., regarding Samuel Cohen
11) Interview with Alice Abrams and Sue Kraus

It should be noted that at the time of my review of these documents Mr. Cohen had passed away and could not be directly assessed. Because of this state of affairs, I have limited the basis of my opinions to the information available from medical records and other collateral sources, and when sufficient data was not present to allow me to provide the court with an opinion with reasonable reliability, I refrained from providing such an opinion.

The records in this case are voluminous, and it is not my intention to discuss aspects of Mr. Cohen's medical condition which are unlikely to have had a direct influence on his testamentary capacity or his ability to resist undue influence. Although I have reviewed all of the records provided to me, I will only address relevant portions of the records in this report.

2/6/03 notes from MCH Health Services (Lynne Bankhead, ARNP). "Short-term memory problems" are noted, and Mr. Cohen is described as a "pleasant but mildly confused 87 yo."

4/22/03 Comprehensive Medical Evaluation, Lynne Bankhead, ARNP. Under Review of Systems, Neuro category, there is a question mark next to memory changes, and under Psyche category depression is circled and "mild" is noted. Under Assessment/Plan it is noted that Mr. Cohen was prescribed Amitriptyline for depression and sleep.

9/29/03 History and Physical performed by William Gross, M.D. Under History of Present Illness, Dr. Gross notes that Mr. Cohen has "some degree of cognitive impairment as well." Under Past Medical History he notes cognitive impairment. Under Family History, Dr. Gross notes that Mr. Cohen was unable to provide any family history due to his cognitive impairment.

9/30/03 Long Pond Healthcare Preadmission Screening. Under Neurological/Cognitive section, the following are noted.

- Mental Status: Alert, Oriented to Place (Not clear if oriented to person or time) and Confused are indicated.
- Memory: Deficits in short and long-term memory are noted.
- Decision Making: Modified Independence is checked.
- Communication: It is noted that his speech is clear but "can be 'halting' grammar errors with wording."
- Emotional Status: Sad, Withdrawn, Cooperative and Pleasant are indicated.

9/30/03 Noncontrast C.T. Evaluation of the Brain, Channing Swan, Radiologist. Conclusion: Normal Noncontrast C.T. Evaluation of the Brain.

10/23/03 Information Sheet, Antidepressant Medications. Notes that Mr. Cohen is taking 10 mg of Celexa daily for mood problems.

10/26/03 Long Pond Healthcare Initial Plan of Care, signed by Dr. Mixon. Under Contradiction/Precautions he notes "fall risk" and "confused." Under Pertinent Medical History "depression with recent start on Celexa." Under Safety Concerns it is noted that he has decreased awareness of deficits and decreased memory. Under Cognition, Impairment is noted.

10/29/03 Minimum Data Set for Nursing Home Resident Assessment and Care Screening, Full Assessment Form.

- Memory: Short-term (5 minutes) memory problems noted, long-term memory okay.
- Memory/Recall Ability: Unable to recall current season, location of own room, staff names/faces, or that he is in a nursing home.
- Ability to Understand Others: Usually understands (may miss some part/content of message) related to cognitive loss/ dementia and communication problems.
- Mood and Behavior Patterns, Verbal expressions of distress (all of the following rated 2, "indicator of this type exhibited daily or almost daily").
    - Resident made negative statements – e.g., "nothing matters; would rather be dead; what is the use; regrets having lived so long; let me die"
    - Repetitive Verbalizations – e.g., calling out for help
    - Repetitive health complaints – e.g., persistently seeks medical attention, obsessive concern with body functions
- Under Resident Assessment Protocol Summary, the following problems were noted: Cognitive Loss, Communication, ADL Functional/Rehabilitation Potential, mood state, activities, falls, nutritional status, pressure ulcers, and psychotropic drug use.

11/18/03 Minimum Data Set for Nursing Home Resident Assessment and Care Screening, Full Assessment Form.

- Memory: Short-term (5 minutes) memory problems noted, long-term memory okay
- Memory Recall Ability: Able to recall current season, and that he is in a nursing home, but cannot recall location of room, staff names, and faces

- Cognitive Skills for Daily Decision-Making: Modified independence – some difficulty in new situations only (related to cognitive loss/dementia)
- Ability to Understand Others: Usually understands (may miss some part/content of message) related to cognitive loss/ dementia and communication problems
- Mood and Behavior Patterns, Verbal expressions of distress (all of the following rated 2, "indicator of this type exhibited daily or almost daily")
  - Resident made negative statements – e.g., "nothing matters; would rather be dead; what is the use; regrets having lived so long; let me die"
  - Repetitive Verbalizations – e.g., calling out for help
  - Repetitive health complaints – e.g., persistently seeks medical attention, obsessive concern with body functions

11/18/03 Interdisciplinary Discharge Plan, Lisa Biedberg, LPN. Notes that Mr. Cohen is oriented, is not confused, and is not combative.

1/29/2004 Green Mountain Community Hospital Emergency Room Consultation, Dr. Mixon. Dr. Mixon notes: "history is obtained from the patient which is somewhat unreliable because of some moderate cognitive impairment."

5/3/04 Consultation, Dr. Alan Thomas. List of current medications includes Celexa (antidepressant) and Aricept (usually given for dementia). Under Assessment/Plan, Pain Control, it is noted that pain seems fairly stable with OxyContin. "Certainly this may cause some confusional problems though. That will need to be watched. Certainly complicated by his history of Alzheimer's type dementia. He is on Aricept."

My review of the medical records in this case raises a number of issues regarding Mr. Cohen's testamentary capacity and the possibility of undue influence in the modification of his will. I will address the issue of testamentary capacity first.

As you are aware, there are a number of components that make up testamentary capacity. The first of these is the ability to understand the nature of the testamentary act. The testator must understand that he is allocating resources and/or property to offspring, relatives, or others. The second component is the ability to understand and recollect his assets and liabilities. It should be noted that this is generally not construed to mean that the testator must have an exact knowledge of his financial situation, but a grossly inaccurate assessment casts doubt on the testator's capacity in this area. The third component involves the testator's knowledge of the natural objects of his bounty, which is taken to mean the ability to understand his relationships with heirs, spouse, parents, and other potential beneficiaries, as well as the impact of the allocation on their situations. Finally, it is generally understood that the person executing the will must be able to keep the first three factors in his mind long enough to make rational choices based on that information.

This case is complicated by the fact that, while a number of physicians and other caregivers noted that Mr. Cohen exhibited a degree of mental confusion some time after the signing of the modified will, there is no evidence of formal assessment of his mental capacities that I could find. There is no evidence that he was ever given a standardized mental status evaluation or a neuropsychological evaluation. Further, it can be difficult to make a differential diagnosis that differentiates the effects of depression from organic factors such as vascular or Alzheimer's type dementia. In this case, Mr. Cohen had suffered a significant loss when his nephew passed away on 9/13/02. As a consequence, the symptoms of mental confusion seen in early 2003 may have been related to depression, dementia, or some combination of the two. In either case, by 9/29/03 Dr. Gross notes that Mr. Cohen is unable to provide a family history due to cognitive impairment. Difficulties recalling family history and the identity of family members would have a direct impact on Mr. Cohen's ability to recall "the natural objects of his bounty," and it is quite possible that he had similar difficulties at the time the new will was executed. Dementia often begins insidiously, and it is likely that if he were noticeably demented in early 2003, he was probably suffering some degree of organic impairment in late 2002. However, it is difficult to know with any precision the extent of any impairment at the time the will was executed. As a consequence, it is my opinion that it is possible that Mr. Cohen lacked testamentary capacity, but it is not possible to state an opinion about this issue to a reasonable degree of psychological certainty.

The issue of possible undue influence will next be considered. As you are aware, undue influence is a more complicated concept than testamentary capacity, and involves the substitution of one person's wishes for another's. In the context of the writing or modification of a will, the testator may, in the abstract, have testamentary capacity, but the wishes of another person are, in fact, what are represented in the will. In the psychological and psychiatric literature a number of indicia of undue influence have been identified. I will list them and provide information about the presence or absence of each of these indicia in this case.

1) The party suspected of exerting undue influence played an active role in procuring the will.

My reading of the deposition of the nephew who was the sole beneficiary of the new will (J.K.) indicates that he was active in obtaining the services of the attorney who drew up the new will, and also arranged for the meetings in which the new will was signed.

2) The individual suspected of exerting undue influence was in a confidential relationship with the testator (e.g., was a close relative or advisor).

Again, it is clearly the case that Mr. Cohen was completely dependent on J.K. and his wife for assistance with activities of daily living, medical care, meal preparation, and transportation.

3) The individual suspected of exerting undue influence profited unduly from the provisions of the will.

Clearly, it is the province of the court to decide whether J.K. benefited unduly from the new will. However, it is important to note that after the death of the nephew with whom Mr. Cohen had resided for many years, J.K. went from modestly benefiting from the provisions of Mr. Cohen's will to becoming the only recipient of his substantial estate.

4) Provisions inconsistent with prior or subsequent expressions of the testator's intentions.

My reading of the material provided to me in this case indicates that throughout his adult life it had been Mr. Cohen's intention to bequeath his estate to the nephew with whom he had resided in the first instance and to his great nieces and nephews in the second. The revised will in this case is clearly inconsistent with Mr. Cohen's long-term prior wishes regarding the disposition of his estate.

5) A relationship between the testator and the beneficiary that created an opportunity to control the testamentary act.

It appears from the material I have reviewed in this case that Mr. Cohen was totally dependent on J.K. and his wife in virtually all aspects of his daily life subsequent to moving in with them. This type of dependency would clearly create an opportunity to control the testamentary act.

6) A mental or physical condition of the testator that facilitates the subversion of the testator's free will.

A review of the available data in this case makes it clear that Mr. Cohen was a shy, anxious, and retiring individual prior to the death of his nephew. It is also clear that he was bereaved and depressed by the unexpected death of his longtime companion, and was left with concerns about how he would have his needs met. The medical records make it clear that medical personnel were noticing cognitive impairment consistent with dementia approximately four months after the signing of the will, and that more significant symptoms of progressive dementia (e.g., memory problems, halting speech, and grammatical errors) were seen by Dr. Gross seven months after that. Clearly, Mr. Cohen was suffering from a number of conditions that would have made him quite vulnerable to undue influence.

Based on the information provided above, it is my opinion that the changes in Mr. Cohen's will were the product of undue influence. His emotional and cognitive problems put him in a vulnerable state, and his total dependence on J.K. and his wife provided the opportunity for the subversion of his free will in the disposition of his estate.

I appreciate the opportunity to perform this assessment. Please feel free to contact me if you require further information or have questions.

Sincerely,

Eric Mart, Ph.D.

Eric G. Mart, Ph.D., ABPP (Forensic)

EGM / km

GLOSSARY

Conservatorship: a judicial authorization for one person to make decisions for another (also called a "guardianship" in some jurisdictions).

Estate: the total of the deceased's assets.

Executor: the person identified in the will as responsible for dispersing the assets of the deceased to the chosen heir(s) (male).

Executrix: the person identified in the will as responsible for dispersing the assets of the deceased to the chosen heir(s) (female).

Guardianship: a judicial authorization for one person to make decisions for another (also called a "conservatorship" in some jurisdictions).

Heirs: the parties who receive the assets of the deceased.

Intestate: where an individual had died without a will, that person is said to have died "intestate."

Natural heirs: the parties who would receive the assets of the deceased if there were no will.

Probate: the judicial procedure where a court disperses the assets of a decedent, often with the assistance of the decedent's will.

Testamentary capacity: the cognitive and emotional capacities necessary to execute a valid will.

Testator: the person (or persons) whose assets are the subject of the will (male).

Testatrix: the person (or persons) whose assets are the subject of the will (female).

Undue influence: where a party has usurped the free will of another.

REFERENCES

CITED REFERENCES

79 Am. Jur. 2d *Wills* § 47 (1964-2009)

79 Am. Jur. 2d *Wills* § 59 (1964-2009)

79 Am. Jur. 2d *Wills* § 60 (1964-2009)

79 Am. Jur. 2d *Wills* § 67 (1964-2009)

79 Am. Jur. 2d *Wills* § 73 (1964-2009)

79 Am. Jur. 2d *Wills* § 75 (1964-2009)

79 Am. Jur. 2d *Wills* § 87 (1964-2009)

79 Am. Jur. 2d *Wills* § 371 (1964-2009)

79 Am. Jur. 2d *Wills* § 374 (1964-2009)

79 Am. Jur. 2d *Wills* § 381 (1964-2009)

American Psychological Association. (2002). *Ethical Principles of Psychologists and Code of Conduct.* Retrieved from http://www.apa.org/ethics/code/code.pdf

American Psychology-Law Society. (2008). *Revision of the Specialty Guidelines for Forensic Psychology*. Retrieved from http://www.ap-ls.org/links/22808sgfp.pdf

Applehans v. Jurgenson, 168 N.E. 327 (Ill. 1929).

Beck, A., Steer, R., & Brown, G. (1996). *Beck Depression Inventory-II.* San Antonio, TX: Pearson.

Ben-Porath, Y. S., & Tellegen, A. (2008). *Minnesota Multiphasic Personality Inventory-2-Restructured Form.* San Antonio, TX: Pearson.

Black's Law Dictionary (2nd pocket ed.). (2001). St. Paul, MN: West Group.

Butcher, J. N., Graham, J., Dahlstrom, W., Tellegen, A., & Kaemmer, B. (1989). *Minnesota Multiphasic Personality Inventory-2: Manual for Administration and Scoring.* Minneapolis, MN: University of Minnesota Press.

Clement v. Rainey, 50 S.W.2d 359 (Tex. Civ. App. 1932).

Cook v. Huff, 552 S.E.2d 83, 85-86 (Ga. 2001).

Coolidge, F. (1999). *Coolidge Assessment Battery.* Port Huron, MI: Sigma Assessment Systems.

De Gale, A. (2003, January 15). Fido can share the wealth [Electronic version]. *The Wichita Eagle*. Retrieved from http://www. kansas.com/MLD/Kansas/news/weird_news/4953297.htm

Delis, D., Kaplan, E., & Kramer, J. (2001). *Delis-Kaplan Executive Function System*. San Antonio, TX: Pearson.

Drogin, E. (2010). *Evaluation for Guardianship*. New York: Oxford University Press.

Frolik, L. A. (1999). Science, common sense, and the determination of mental capacity. *Psychology, Public Policy & Law, 5*(1), 41-58.

Grisso, T. (2003). *Evaluating Competencies: Forensic Assessments and Instruments* (2nd ed.). New York: Kluwer Academic/Plenum.

Grisso T., & Appelbaum P. S. (1995). The MacArthur treatment competence study. III: Abilities of patients to consent to psychiatric and medical treatment. *Law and Human Behavior, 19*(2), 149-174.

Gudjonsson, G. (1987). *Gudjonsson Suggestibility Scales*. London: Psychology Press.

Hamilton v. Morgan, 112 So. 80, 82 (Fla. 1927).

Hatheway v. Smith, 65 A. 1058, 1060 (Conn. 1907).

Holmes v. Campbell College, 125 P. 25, 26 (Kan. 1926).

In re Brzowsky's Estate, 67 N.W.2d 384 (Wis. 1954).

In re Estate of Anderson, 246 N.W.2d 586, 587 (Neb. 1976).

In re Estate of Bennett, 865 P.2d 1062, 1076 (Kan. App. 1993).

In re Estate of Congdon, 309 N.W.2d 261 (Minn. 1981).

In re Estate of Kesler, 702 P.2d 86, 96 (Utah 1985).

In re Estate of Raney, 799 P.2d 986 (Kan. 1990).

In re Kleeb's Estate, 320 N.W.2d 459 (Neb. 1982).

In re Sixkiller, 32 P.2d 936 (Oakl. 1934).

Jackson, D. (1988). *Basic Personality Inventory*. Port Huron, MI: Sigma Assessment Systems.

Jurica, P., Leitten, C., & Mattis, S. (2001). *Dementia Rating Scale-2 Professional Manual*. Lutz, FL: Psychological Assessment Resources.

Kaufman, A. S., & Kaufman, N. L. (2004). *Kaufman Brief Intelligence Test (KBIT-2) Manual* (2nd ed.). Bloomington, MN: Pearson Assessments.

Kendrick-Owens v. Clanton, 524 S.E.2d 237, 238 (Ga. 1999).

Madden v. Cornett, 160 S.W.2d. 607, 611 (Ky. App. 1942).

Marson, D. C., Huthwaite, J. C., & Hebert, K. (2004). Testamentary capacity and undue influence in the elderly: A jurisprudent therapy perspective. *Law & Psychology Review, 28*, 71-87.

Melton, G. B., Petrila, J., Poythress, N. G., & Slobogin, C. (2007). *Psychological Evaluations for the Courts: A Handbook for Mental Health Professionals and Lawyers* (3rd ed.). New York: Guilford.

Morey, L. C. (1991). *Personality Assessment Inventory*. Odessa, FL: Psychological Assessment Resources.

Pape v. Byrd, 582 N.E.2d.164, 168 (Ill. 1991).

Perr, I. N. (1981). Wills, testamentary capacity and undue influence. *Bulletin of the American Academy of Psychiatry and the Law, 9,* 15-22.

Powell, D., Kaplan, E., Whitla, D., Weintraub, S., Catlin, R., & Funkenstein, H. (2004). *MicroCog: Assessment of Cognitive Functioning.* San Antonio, TX: Pearson.

Pyle v. Sayers, 39 S.W.3d 774, 778 (Ark. 2001).

Randolph, C. (1998). *Repeatable Battery for the Assessment of Neuropsychological Status.* San Antonio, TX: Pearson.

Reitan, R. M., & Wolfson, D. (1993). *The Halstead-Reitan Neuropsychological Test Battery: Theory and Clinical Interpretation.* Tucson, AZ: Neuropsychology Press.

Reynolds, C., & Kamphaus, R. (1998). *Reynolds Intellectual Assessment Scales and the Reynolds Intellectual Screening Test.* Lutz, FL: Psychological Assessment Resources.

Rogers, R. (2001). *Handbook of Diagnostic and Structured Interviewing.* New York: Guilford Press.

Schinka, J. A. (1988). *Mental Status Checklist for Adults.* Lutz, FL: Psychological Assessment Resources.

Schmidt, M. (1996). *Rey Auditory Verbal Learning Test: A Handbook.* Los Angeles, CA: Western Psychological Services.

Sheslow, D., & Adams, W. (2003). *Wide Range Assessment of Memory and Learning (Second Edition) Administration and Technical Manual.* Lutz, FL: Psychological Assessment Resources.

Shulman, K., & Feinstein, A. (2003). *Quick Cognitive Screening for Clinicians: Mini Mental, Clock-Drawing and Other Brief Tests.* London: Taylor & Francis.

Simon, R. I., & Shuman, D. W. (Eds.). (2002). *Retrospective Assessment of Mental States in Litigation: Predicting the Past.* Washington, DC: American Psychiatric Publishing.

Singelmann v. Singelmann, 548 S.E.2d 343, 346 (Ga. 2001).

Slaughter v. Heath, 57 S.E. 69, 71 (Ga. 1907).

Smith v. Vice, 641 So. 2d 785 (Ala. 1984).

Spar, J. E., & Garb, A. S. (1992). Assessing competency to make a will. *American Journal of Psychiatry, 149*(2), 169-174.

Stern, R. A., & White, T. (2003). *Neuropsychological Assessment Battery.* Lutz, FL: Psychological Assessment Resources.

Wechsler, D. (1997). *Wechsler Memory Scale III.* San Antonio, TX: Pearson.

Wechsler, D. (1999). *Wechsler Abbreviated Scale of Intelligence.* San Antonio, TX: Pearson.

Wechsler, D. (2008). *Wechsler Adult Intelligence Scale* (4th ed.). San Antonio, TX: Pearson.

Wiley, J. (2001). *TheraForms.* Retrieved from http://www.wiley.com/legacy/products/subject/psychology/theraforms/index.htm

Winter v. American Parkinson's Disease Association, 85 N.Y.2d 715, 720 (N.Y. 1995).

Wong, J. G., Clare, I. C. H., Holland, A. J., Watson, P. C., & Gunn, M. (2000). The capacity of people with a 'mental disability' to make a health care decision. *Psychological Medicine, 30*(2), 295-306.

Zorn v. Zorn, 64 S.W.2d 626 (Mo. 1933).

CITED INSTRUMENTS AND ORDERING INFORMATION

Basic Personality Inventory (BPI)
Sigma Assessment Systems
P.O. Box 610757
Port Huron, MI 48061-0757
Phone: 800-265-1285
Fax: 800-361-9411
www.sigmaassessmentsystems.com

Beck Depression Inventory-II (BDI-II)
Pearson Assessments
19500 Bulverde Road
San Antonio, TX 78259-3701
Phone: 800-627-7271
Fax: 800-232-1223
www.pearsonassessments.com

Coolidge Assessment Battery (CAB)
Sigma Assessment Systems
P.O. Box 610757
Port Huron, MI 48061-0757
Phone: 800-265-1285
Fax: 800-361-9411
www.sigmaassessmentsystems.com

Delis-Kaplan Executive Function System (D-KEFS)
Pearson Assessments
19500 Bulverde Road
San Antonio, TX 78259-3701
Phone: 800-627-7271
Fax: 800-232-1223
www.pearsonassessments.com

Dementia Rating Scale-2 Professional Manual (DRS-2)
Psychological Assessment Resources, Inc.
16204 N. Florida Avenue
Lutz, FL 33549
Phone: 800-331-8378
Fax: 800-727-9329
www.parinc.com

Gudjonsson Suggestibility Scales (GSS)
Psychology Press/Taylor & Francis, Inc.
7625 Empire Drive
Florence, KY 41042-2919
Phone: 800-634-7064
Fax: 800-248-4724
www.psypress.com

The Halstead-Reitan Neuropsychological Test Battery
Reitan Neuropsychology Lab
PO Box 66080
Tucson, AZ 85728-6080
Phone: 520-577-2970
Fax: 520-577-2940
www.reitanlabs.com

Kaufman Brief Intelligence Test Second Edition (KBIT-2)
Pearson Assessments
19500 Bulverde Road
San Antonio, TX 78259-3701
Phone: 800-627-7271
Fax: 800-232-1223
www.pearsonassessments.com

Mental Status Checklist for Adults
Psychological Assessment Resources, Inc.
16204 N. Florida Avenue
Lutz, FL 33549
Phone: 800-331-8378
Fax: 800-727-9329
www.parinc.com

MicroCog: Assessment of Cognitive Functioning
Pearson Assessments
19500 Bulverde Road
San Antonio, TX 78259-3701
Phone: 800-627-7271
Fax: 800-232-1223
www.pearsonassessments.com

Minnesota Multiphasic Personality Inventory-2 (MMPI-2)
Pearson Assessments
19500 Bulverde Road
San Antonio, TX 78259-3701
Phone: 800-627-7271
Fax: 800-232-1223
www.pearsonassessments.com

Minnesota Multiphasic Personality Inventory-2-Restructured Form (MMPI-2-RF)
Pearson Assessments
19500 Bulverde Road
San Antonio, TX 78259-3701
Phone: 800-627-7271
Fax: 800-232-1223
www.pearsonassessments.com

Neuropsychological Assessment Battery (NAB)
Psychological Assessment Resources, Inc.
16204 N. Florida Avenue
Lutz, FL 33549
Phone: 800-331-8378
Fax: 800-727-9329
www.parinc.com

Personality Assessment Inventory (PAI)
Psychological Assessment Resources, Inc.
16204 N. Florida Avenue
Lutz, FL 33549
Phone: 800-331-8378
Fax: 800-727-9329
www.parinc.com

Repeatable Battery for the Assessment of Neuropsychological Status (RBANS)
Pearson Assessments
19500 Bulverde Road
San Antonio, TX 78259-3701
Phone: 800-627-7271
Fax: 800-232-1223
www.pearsonassessments.com

Rey Auditory Verbal Learning Test (RAVLT)
Western Psychological Services
12031 Wilshire Boulevard
Los Angeles, CA 90025-1251
Phone: 800-648-8857
Fax: 310-478-7838
www.wpspublish.com

Reynolds Intellectual Assessment Scales (RAIS) and the Reynolds Intellectual Screening Test (RIST)
Psychological Assessment Resources, Inc.
16204 N. Florida Avenue
Lutz, FL 33549
Phone: 800-331-8378
Fax: 800-727-9329
www.parinc.com

TheraForms
www.wiley.com/legacy/products/subject/psychology/theraforms/index.htm

Wechsler Abbreviated Scale of Intelligence (WASI)
Pearson Assessments
19500 Bulverde Road
San Antonio, TX 78259-3701
Phone: 800-627-7271
Fax: 800-232-1223
www.pearsonassessments.com

Wechsler Adult Intelligence Scale – Fourth Edition (WAIS-IV)
Pearson Assessments
19500 Bulverde Road
San Antonio, TX 78259-3701
Phone: 800-627-7271
Fax: 800-232-1223
www.pearsonassessments.com

Wechsler Memory Scale III – Third Edition (WMS-III)
Pearson Assessments
19500 Bulverde Road
San Antonio, TX 78259-3701
Phone: 800-627-7271
Fax: 800-232-1223
www.pearsonassessments.com

Wide Range Assessment of Memory and Learning, Second Edition (WRAML2)
Psychological Assessment Resources, Inc.
16204 N. Florida Avenue
Lutz, FL 33549
Phone: 800-331-8378
Fax: 800-727-9329
www.parinc.com

INTRODUCTION TO THE CD-ROM

CD-ROM INFORMATION

The material on the CD-ROM is saved as Adobe Portable Document Format (PDF) files. In order to use this material, you will need to have *Adobe Reader* or other software capable of reading Adobe Portable Document Format (PDF) files installed on your computer. See "System Requirements" for information on how you can obtain a free copy of *Adobe Reader*.

TABLE OF CONTENTS OF THE CD-ROM

Montreal Cognitive Assessment (***MoCA***)
  Administration and Scoring
  Instrument
  Normative Data
  References
Semi-Structured Interview for the Assessment of
    Testamentary Capacity (***SSIATC***)

SYSTEM REQUIREMENTS

If you have *Adobe Reader* installed on your computer, this CD-ROM may be used with most versions of the Windows operating system as well as most versions of other operating systems. A free version of *Adobe Reader* may be downloaded at the *Adobe Reader* website:

http://www.adobe.com/products/reader

That site also contains detailed information about system requirements for using the software, a downloadable user's guide, user's forums, and other useful information. Most users find that simply downloading the software enables them to open and use PDF files such as those included on the CD-ROM.

HOW TO INSTALL AND USE THE FILES

After *Adobe Reader* is installed, you can copy the contents of the CD-ROM to a convenient place on your hard disk and each file should open automatically when you click on it. You can identify Adobe Portable Document Format files because they all have a PDF extension (e.g., Sample.pdf). If Windows asks you to choose a program to open the file with, choose Adobe Reader's latest version.

Adobe Reader allows you to print exact reproductions of the material on the CD-ROM to whatever printer(s) are installed on your computer;

however, it will not allow you to edit or modify the materials. If you want to edit or modify the material, you will need to order one of Adobe's other products from www.adobe.com.

PERMISSION TO USE THIS MATERIAL

Purchasers of *The Practical Assessment of Testamentary Capacity and Undue Influence in the Elderly* have an unlimited right to print copies of the materials on the CD-ROM for use with their clients. However, they may not share copies of either this CD-ROM or the materials contained herein with others without explicit written consent from the publisher, Professional Resource Exchange, Inc. (PO Box 3197, Sarasota, FL 34230-3197)

If You Found This Book Useful . . .

You might want to know more about our other titles.

If you would like to receive our latest catalog, please return this form:

Name: ______________________________
(Please Print)

Address: ______________________________

Address: ______________________________

City/State/Zip: ______________________________
This is ❒ home ❒ office

Telephone: (__________)______________________________

E-mail: ______________________________

Fax: (__________) ______________________________

I am a:

❒ Psychologist	❒ Mental Health Counselor
❒ Psychiatrist	❒ Marriage and Family Therapist
❒ Attorney	❒ Not in Mental Health Field
❒ Clinical Social Worker	❒ Other: ______________

◆ ◆ ◆

Professional Resource Press
P.O. Box 3197
Sarasota, FL 34230-3197

Telephone: 800-443-3364
FAX: 941-343-9201
E-mail: orders@prpress.com
Website: http://www.prpress.com

PATC/8/10

Add A Colleague To Our Mailing List . . .

If you would like us to send our latest catalog to one of your colleagues, please return this form:

Name: ____

(Please Print)

Address: ____

Address: ____

City/State/Zip: ______________________________________

This is ❒ home ❒ office

Telephone: (__________)________________________________

E-mail: ____

Fax: (__________) ____________________________________

This person is a:

❒ Psychologist
❒ Psychiatrist
❒ Attorney
❒ Clinical Social Worker
❒ Mental Health Counselor
❒ Marriage and Family Therapist
❒ Not in Mental Health Field
❒ Other: ____________________

Name of person completing this form: ____________________

◆ ◆ ◆

Professional Resource Press
P.O. Box 3197
Sarasota, FL 34230-3197

Telephone: 800-443-3364
FAX: 941-343-9201
E-mail: orders@prpress.com
Website: http://www.prpress.com